Cancer changes everything; but having someone in your life, who understands, changes the journey. Let this first hand account of a walk with cancer be that change for you.

—Shanna Decker, Cancer Survivor /Amputee, Motivational Speaker, Seven–Time National Award Winner for Volunteerism.

Time Out

Time Out

A Family's Journey of Faith
and Hope through Childhood Cancer

David A. Kelly

TATE PUBLISHING & Enterprises

Scripture quotations marked "NIV" are taken from the *Holy Bible, New International Version* ®, Copyright © 1973, 1978, 1984 by International Bible Society. Used by permission of Zondervan Publishing House. All rights reserved.

This novel is a work of nonfiction. The names, descriptions, entities, and incidents included in the story are based on the lives of real people.

The opinions expressed by the author are not necessarily those of Tate Publishing, LLC.

Published by Tate Publishing & Enterprises, LLC
127 E. Trade Center Terrace | Mustang, Oklahoma 73064 USA
1.888.361.9473 | www.tatepublishing.com

Tate Publishing is committed to excellence in the publishing industry. The company reflects the philosophy established by the founders, based on Psalm 68:11,
"The Lord gave the word and great was the company of those who published it."

Book design copyright © 2009 by Tate Publishing, LLC. All rights reserved.
Cover design by Blake Brasor
Interior design by Lindsay B. Behrens

Published in the United States of America

ISBN: 978-1-60799-619-4
1. Biography & Autobiography / Medical   2. Health & Fitness / Diseases / Cancer
09.07.07

Dedication

This book is dedicated to Hannah Jane. You continue to inspire and amaze us.

Acknowledgments

It is with great privilege and gratitude to have the opportunity to write this book on behalf of all those who have experienced a child going through cancer. Thanks to God, our Lord and Savior, for giving us the strength, mercy, and grace to make this walk.

To my awesome daughter, Hannah, who led the way in faith and showed us all what courage looks like. She continues to be a measure of strength and fearlessness for our family.

To my beautiful, loving, and supportive wife, Kim. If it weren't for her encouragement to share this daily journey, our story would have been a memory of chemo poles, shots, and hospital rooms. Instead, it's a testament to the grace of God and to all those children who battle cancer.

To our boys, Sam and Max, who kept their focus on the importance of faith and family. They stayed strong for us when all of our focus needed to be on Hannah. As we came to learn, the siblings of a child afflicted with cancer are hurting more often then they let on because of their need to stay strong.

To the tremendous work of the medical profession that lifts spirits and brings hope along with medical aid to those who battle cancer. You are truly a blessing to every family you touch. The number one thing I remember most is when we were told by a physician, "I don't deal in percentages. Percentages don't tell you anything. I deal in the child and his/her strength and ability to get through it."

To our family and friends, who stood beside us and held us up in prayer. What a tremendous gift you have given our family. It's been one giant wrapping of your arms around us, to hold us up and move us forward.

Table of Contents

Prologue

It was December of 1996 when we first noticed that our newborn, Hannah, had a fullness in her right wrist, her little baby fingernails pressing into her palm like razors against the skin. "Have you noticed this?" My wife, Kim, pointed out Hannah's then strange lump. We took a closer look and discovered a redness sitting on a small bump just below the wrist.

The next day we scheduled the appointment with our local pediatrician, who quickly referred us to the University of Chicago and a specialist dealing with what was believed to be a hemangioma (a grouping of blood vessels).

Two years of trips back and forth to Chicago under monitored care became a bit of a joke to me. It was as simple as predicting the forecast on a summer morning—*today will be warm with clear skies*. I already had the routine of the doctor down pat ... "Good morning. How is Hannah today? Great, great. The mass seems to be growing along with her. She looks very healthy. I'll see you in six months. Any questions?"

By the time Hannah turned two, our last trip to this doctor took on a whole new feel. "Let's schedule a biopsy and see what's in there," the doctor told us without the typical script. "I have a good friend of mine who's in charge at the Children's Hospital of Chicago. I've already talked to him and he's aware of Hannah's situation."

Pre–surgery for the biopsy went well—which is to say, watching your two–year–old laying on a big hospital bed as she's wheeled away places your heart directly in the middle, upper portion of your throat. As the surgery began, we were led to the parent waiting room where everyone had the same glazed–over expression. It was a room waiting to exhale. As the doctors began coming into the room, one–by–one they would find their perspective parents and give them the good news. "Surgery went well, and he/she is in recovery at the moment. You'll be able to go be with your child shortly."

We waited for our doctor to show up through the magical door of good news. *Ahhhh, finally!* "Mr. and Mrs. Kelly, would you like to follow me into this other room?" His facial expression was not the same as the others who had preceded him. *What's the "other" room, and why hasn't anybody else been invited there?* My stomach hit the high cycle of a washing machine. As we sat down, we were joined by a nurse who quietly and politely shut the door behind her. I remember the look on her face as the doctor explained that the biopsy went well, but he felt that Hannah had cancer based on all the cases he had seen. "The pathologist must still determine this, but I have seen a number of cases, and the tissue we took is very similar to cancer."

The nurse reached across from her seat to comfort Kim, who I believe was crying by now. I went into shock as I sat there thinking that this was supposed to be a simple, unusual grouping of blood vessels, not cancer! I couldn't help but think about the past two years of travel to Chicago, all the while allowing this cancer to grow inside her and not doing a darn thing.

The last thing I remember from that day is the doctor getting up to leave and telling us, "You have this room as long as you need it." I didn't want the room; I wanted my daughter! I wanted this to be something simple, something fixable, and something that wouldn't have the word *cancer* in it.

I stood at the end of Hannah's bed in the recovery room watching her as she slept off the anesthesia. Many thoughts were racing through my mind. The doctor had told us that he felt it was a fibrosarcoma. *What the heck is a fi–bro–sarcoma?* I knew one thing was for sure ... I was going to get on the Internet and find out everything possible about this cancer.

"Whatever you do, do not get on the Internet and begin looking this cancer up," a voice came from behind me. I turned to see the recovery room nurse. *How did she know what I was thinking?* "The Internet is full of page after page of information, and it's really too early to get yourself worked up over something that hasn't been determined yet. Besides, the Internet information has nothing you want to see. It will just scare you even more." The nurse was trying to comfort us as much as she could. I'm sure panic, fear, disbelief, and more fear had been written all over our faces.

Over the next two weeks, we prayed, cried, and prayed some more. The diagnosis from the pathologist came back and was positive for cancer, but they also said it was a difficult read, so they were sending it to a lab in California for a second look. *A second look? Are these people trying to send me into a mental breakdown? Let's move forward and cut this thing out!*

During these weeks, we were introduced to the term *oncologist*. "We're sending you to speak with an oncologist. You can have a seat in the waiting room while I set that up," the nurse told us as we stood waiting at the office counter. *What the heck is an oncologist, and why would I need to see one of those?* The oncology department ended up sending a resident to the pediatric floor who explained that he was not the oncologist that we would be working with, but would go over any questions we might have.

The fundamental problem when you enter into the cancer world for the first time is an age–old problem: You don't know what questions to ask because you don't know anything. I suppose the same can be said of the mechanical world. If anything goes wrong, I find myself standing beside a mechanic as I stare blankly into the engine wondering what the heck is making such an awful noise.

When you hear the words that your child has cancer, the first thing you want to do (aside from vomiting) is to have it removed. It seemed like over the course of two weeks, things were going slower and slower…then a lot slower than we had hoped. I had been told too many times to go home and wait for a call. "The doctor is tied up right now, and we have no idea how long he will be. Go home for now and we'll call you later."

We made the decision to pack up and head to the Mayo Clinic. Gathering documentation was a bit tougher than I had thought it would be. I started at the pediatric floor with, "Hi, I'm here to let you know that we've decided to take our daughter and go to the Mayo Clinic. Our hometown pediatrician has already made the call, and they are expecting us."

"Does the doctor know you are leaving?" the lady at the desk asked, taking a tone with me.

"Probably not." I didn't want confrontation; I wanted records. The people at Mayo had told us to bring records and MRI scans with us. "Well, you'll need to talk with him," she said as she picked up the phone.

Great. Now I have to go through the uncomfortable feeling of making a nice doctor feel bad. Wait a second! This is our daughter, and we're not just sitting around anymore.

We ended up having the meeting and getting the records released. It was a bit uncomfortable, but the doctor was very pleasant and understood that we were anxious to move forward—which wasn't happening.

At Mayo, we arrived in the dead of the night, slept very little, and awoke the next morning ready to find out what was happening with Hannah. We didn't have our scans on hand as we were supposed to because the hospital in Chicago couldn't locate her MRI scans (but assured us they would send them on to Mayo when they did). We were hoping that this wouldn't slow the process down any.

That day we met with a group of doctors from pediatric oncology, pediatric orthopedics, and pediatric surgery. Their response to our missing scans was, "That's okay, we want to get our own anyway. Those were just to compare." So we took more MRI scans and a few other tests. The doctors told us, "We'll meet tomorrow to go over the results. We have our pathology department looking at the biopsy right now." We had grown tired of holding our breath. We met with all the doctors once again. They told us, "Hannah has a tumor, but it's not cancerous. Our pathologist said it was a difficult diagnosis, but it's not cancer. It's classified as a fibromatosis." The lead oncologist explained that Hannah had a fibrous tumor that would grow like a vine, wrapping itself around muscle, tendons, and ligaments. She said that it may or may not cause handicapping when it came to movement in her arm, and it typically becomes smaller over time before dissolving into the body.

That was Hannah at two-years-old. From that point we made the journey to Mayo every other year to monitor her progress.

1998–MRI scans show mass just above the wrist extending to just below the elbow.

1999–MRI scan shows mass retracting slightly.

2001–MRI scan suggests mass is smaller.

2003–MRI scans show a continued decrease in the tumor mass.

2005–MRI scans show the mass remaining the same size.

2007–scheduled trip in August … we never made it that long.

What you are about to read was written as a series of blog entries with a few personal journal entries added. Leaving the support of friends and family at home, we journeyed to the Mayo Clinic in Minnesota—removed from family and friends. Through the use of a blog site, we not only were able to keep our connection, but also recounted our story as we weaved through childhood cancer.

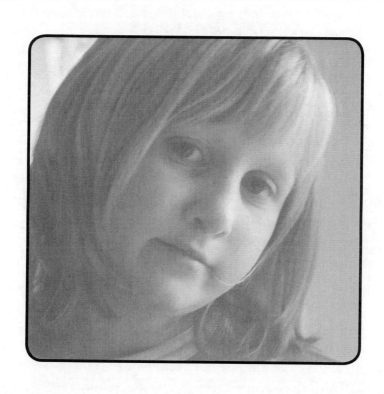

2007 April

Hello, God?

Just this past week, Hannah, my ten–year–old daughter, finished a terrific junior travel basketball season by wrapping up an 18–6 record and celebrating with her fellow teammates. Two hours after the end of season basketball bash, we're sitting in the emergency room because of a rather large lump on her right forearm, which already hosted a nasty benign tumor, had popped up and was causing pain. It sure puts a winning basketball season in perspective quickly and makes you realize what the important things in life really are. Ten hours beyond the emergency room visit, we were on our way to the Mayo Clinic in Rochester, Minnesota, for more tests and hopefully some answers.

You do a great deal of talking with God when you're in crisis mode. I wasn't really talking to him a whole lot during the basketball celebration, but he and I had a direct line of communication as I made my way to the hospital and from Michigan to Mayo.

Strength, mercy, and grace were the top three things for which I prayed. When something like this strikes, it's one thing to be prepared and to take the right steps, but it's another thing to turn it over in prayer.

I prayed not only for my daughter, but also for my students. As a teacher, I like to be the guy in the room and not get too emotional with the kids, but I do pray that things are going well for them. I pray that my fourth grade students have the strength to handle the change in class while I'm away, show mercy on a new teacher as she gets to know them and they her, and the grace to show what wonderful kids they are. I know that prayers are being given on behalf of my daughter, and we are truly blessed for that alone.

So for those kids that are reading this, take care of one another, be kind, and I will be back soon.

Hello, God? I heard there were lightning bolts in Michigan on Thursday—hope they weren't aimed in the direction of my class.

> And the prayer offered in faith will make the sick
> person well; the Lord will raise him up.
> James 5:15 (NIV)

May

Exploration

Everything revolves around the biopsy. Doctor Shives, who has been with us since the first diagnosis of fibro-mitosis, did the biopsy this morning. They typically schedule children early in the morning because they know parents are so impatient—and children are a special priority. I'm guessing the latter is truer.

Dr. Shives came to talk to us regarding the surgery and what they found. I had a flashback from Chicago, eight years earlier, when the doctor came out of the very first biopsy Hannah had. "Mr. and Mrs. Kelly? Would you please step into this room?" It was in that tiny room where we first heard the words, "We believe your daughter has cancer." It's at a point like this that you become numb to the world around you, and you want to call for a timeout, stopping everything dead in its tracks and rewinding life until you reach normal again.

Dr. Thomas Shives is the expert when it comes to tumor removal at the Mayo Clinic in Rochester. Yet, through his biopsy, he was cautious to not stake his claims on what he thought it might be. Instead he explained that the surgery went very well and that Hannah would be brought back to us in the recovery room shortly. With a confident smile on his face, he turned and walked out. Dr. Shives always has a confident smile, though, so it was difficult to read what the growth might be.

When You Just Listen

Day 1:

Days passed since Dr. Shives biopsied Hannah. We were waiting for our turn to speak with Dr. Vilmarie Rodriguez, our pediatric oncology doctor, and to hear the results. As a parent, waiting to hear what your child may or may not have is nothing short of pure torture. Every breath you take is a deep one that requires a slow exhale...you don't want to give away the fact that you're scared, anxious, and on the brink of losing it all together. After all, I'm the dad. I'm supposed to be strong for the rest of us.

Dr. Rodriguez entered the room with a doorknob in one hand and a stack of charts in the other. "Hannah has cancer." She said it plainly without hesitation.

Time froze as jumbled thoughts flashed through my mind as she made her way across the room to her desk and chair. *What does this mean? Boy, I'm glad she didn't hold back. Cancer is not what we had prayed for. How could she just open the door and blurt something out like that? Can we schedule the operation to remove it today? What are the statistics on children with cancer? I won't lose my daughter.*

While I didn't appreciate hearing those words, I was relieved that she didn't go into it slowly. It was like ripping the Band–Aid right off. Had she done the hand–holding, soft–voice routine as she attempted to tell us the news, I would have been miserable.

Once Dr. Rodriguez was seated, she immediately began telling us the steps that we would take in order to rid Hannah of the cancer. It was difficult to even look at Hannah, who sat between Kim and me. I kept my focus on what the doctor was saying, but I could hear the emotion in Kim as she fought back tears.

Dr. Rodriguez must have been a pro at this by now—the breaking of this kind of news. The Mayo Clinic, after all, must see hundreds of children a year who make the trek with their families to get some of the best care around. As she rattled off the protocol for treatment, I heard Hannah whisper gently to Kim, "It will be okay, Mom."

I don't imagine that the lump in my throat could have gotten any bigger than when I listened to my ten–year–old reassure us. That's the strength of faith. That's the strength of a child. That's Hannah.

> I pray that out of his glorious riches he may strengthen you with power through his Spirit in your inner being, so that Christ may dwell in your hearts through faith. And I pray that love, may have power, together with all the saints, to grasp how wide and long and high and deep is the love of Christ, and to know this love that surpasses knowledge—that you may be filled to the measure of all the fullness of God.
>
> Ephesians 3:16–19 (NIV)

Stick, Prod, Poke, Scan

Day 2 (morning):
In the midst of all the testing, there's one thing that I've realized—Wi–Fi is an excellent thing. Some very good friends lent me their laptop with Wi–Fi. With the availability of their computer and Wi–Fi, I can connect to everyone back home who look for intentional prayers on behalf of Hannah. Through those who are praying we are in God's hands. This goes beyond the good hands of the wonderful doctors we have at Mayo. Today proved to be a great deal of data collecting. The doctors had us all over the downtown area visiting various offices for more and more ... and more tests. The best way to finish a day like this was with a lot of swimming back at our hotel.

I was up early due to a humming noise outside. It seems that the restaurant next to our hotel is having all of its carpets cleaned as a team of vans are parked at every restaurant entrance possible.

Today is planning day. We will find out the results of all the tests from yesterday as well as what the overall plan for Hannah will be. Have you ever not wanted to be told something, but at the same time you can't wait? That sums up the day we're about to have.

Tests Looking Good

Day 2 (afternoon):

Good news today. The tests show no spreading of the cancer. The doctor did say that this tumor is so rare that it's being closely studied by the National Group of Oncology. Her treatment begins tomorrow. For today, our spirits have been lifted as prayers are answered by the cancer not spreading beyond her right forearm. We will have about two weeks after we return home to prepare for a summer away. Our prayers continue to be for no spreading, but also include the medicine (chemo) doing its job on the tumor. The doctor did say that most cancers will shrink as a response to the drugs, but that there is a chance that the tumor may not. We are choosing to remain focused on the positive and think *shrink*.

The Port

Day 3:

The port is a small, spaceship–looking, stainless steel piece with a gel bubble in the middle. It has a small flexible tube attached to it. The port rests under the skin (so all you see is a small bump), and the tube runs to a vein above the heart. The tube is held in place by the suction of the blood as it is pulled toward the heart. Once in place, it shouldn't move at all.

When the doctors need to inject anything in Hannah, they will do it through the port. This allows for fewer needles as a multitude of medicine will be given through an IV, and it's easier access when compared to poking around for a vein. The port has to be surgically installed, so a day in the hospital is normal.

Anesthesia is given through a mask. Hannah got to choose from an assortment of flavors to breathe in. She chose bubble gum (a real stretch for any kid). Sure enough, I got to go into the operating room with her until she fell asleep, and the room smelled just like bubble gum. As she breathed deep, the doctor told her a story of a magical candy store. We need to get this guy in for story–time at the school. She received her IV after she fell asleep. Then I left to go back to the waiting room.

Coming out of anesthesia is like trying to wake up from a deep sleep. Only you don't have Mom and Dad yelling at you to get up. So, you get to go back to sleep and dream away—probably dreaming of some magical candy store. As the doctor explained it, time freezes for you while you're under, but your parents' time doubles to take up the slack. The patient always feels like the whole thing just took a second, while for parents an hour seems like two hours. That doctor is a very wise man.

According to the medical staff, your side feels sore for about a day or two with a port. Some people have trouble lifting their arms because the skin moves, and they feel it pull. I would imagine it's like bad sunburn—when you move, it hurts. So you have to lay still and suffer with watching cartoon after cartoon, unless you choose to watch a favorite movie. The hospital has a "movie on demand" program. Each room has a thick book of movie listings. All you do is pick one—that's the hard part.

Day three winds down. Tomorrow is the beginning of the treatment.

Motorcycles Are Coming

Day 4:
Treatment has begun and the medicine seems to interchange and to flow from the metal pole like cars going through the oil change line. Once one bag is empty, another is hung, and the drip begins flowing from start.

I'm learning that there are a number of medicines. For example, just to kick things off today, Hannah was given a medicine to combat an upset stomach. It seems that as the potent medicines move through her body to combat any and everything, she may feel a bit sick to her stomach. Well, after a long day, I'm happy to report that her first medicine worked.

The nurse told us that some kids don't get sick, while others just take longer to have the sickness develop. Tomorrow will tell.

Hannah's biggest issue today was all the visitors. Doctors in teams rotated through the room. If you were a big fan of *West Wing*, where the group constantly walked the White House corridors in a herd, then you have a good mental picture of the doctors at Saint Mary's Hospital. Hannah has been seen by the oncology group, who work at fighting the cancer; the surgical group, who will later operate to take the tumor out; the nutritionist who gave us the news that it's calories first, then proteins, followed by carbohydrates and vegetables in the list of importance for Hannah's health.

The clergy, who we consider to be the first defense of Hannah's well–being, stopped by to lift us up in spirit and faith. There's nothing more powerful than God's grace and mercy. Of course, in between all the groups dropping by for a visit or checkup was the nursing staff. These wonderful people kept feeding us with more and more information on what to expect and how to best care for Hannah. The final visit of the day came from her brothers and grandparents, who had made the trip to be with her as she begins this long road. With all this action, Hannah was spent by early evening.

Tomorrow should be a fun day. A motorcycle charity ride finishes its route right in front of the hospital. It's a good thing I brought my camera!

For the Children—In the News

Day 5:

Starting over ... the first round of medicine was completed throughout the night, and we began with the order of treatment all over again. As the first order of business this morning, the non–vomit medicine was administered to Hannah. I really should get some of this stuff for school as many times as I hear kids say, "Mr. Kelly, I think I'm going to ... " So far, so good as we roll into the early evening.

Today we had the motorcycle ride wrap up at the hospital where a check was presented to the Mayo Eugenio Litta Children's Hospital. The motorcycles were lined up on one side of the parking lot, while tables loaded with food lined the other side. In the middle of it all were the news people, bikers, patients, and hospital staff. Hannah had to be accompanied by a nurse as she strolled the lot with her metal stand, all the while receiving her medicine as it dripped down into the tubes and through the port into her body.

A purple bike in the middle caught her eye, and the staff was quick to help her aboard. What followed next was completely unexpected. She was photographed and a news camera lady asked to interview her for the evening news. It was really cool, except for the fact that my bike was not present to sit among the other chrome wonders. As the dad, I too was interviewed—good thing I had one on of my Harley shirts. It would be shocking if I didn't.

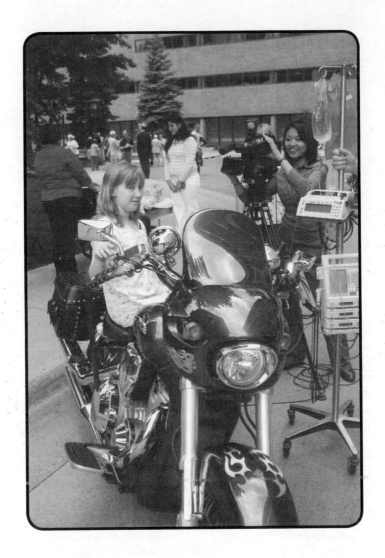

Unfortunately it wasn't *Dateline* or national evening news coverage, so the interview stayed local. Who would have thought that Hannah would be interviewed in her pajamas, sitting on top of a motorcycle, in the middle of a parking lot, surrounded by bikers, while receiving a chemo treatment?

We didn't spend much time after that mingling and eating because Hannah gets tired rather quickly, so back to the room we came. In for the night, another day down.

Toxic What?

Day 6:

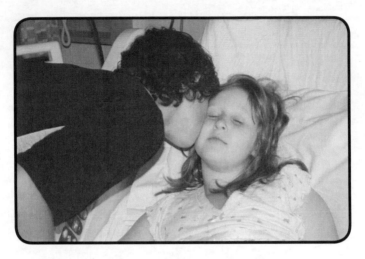

It's the last day of treatment. It's like being in a marathon race. You can see the finish line, and it's all downhill. As the nurse walked into the room dressed in her all–blue smock garb and rubber gloves (to protect her from the toxic meds), she announced loudly, "Last one!" To which Hannah replied, "Oh good." You could feel her relief.

Today went by really slowly—maybe because it was Sunday and it's meant to be a day of rest and peace, or maybe it was because her body is reaching the point of being worn down; and therefore, she slept most of the day.

Hannah's appetite dropped off quite a bit as well today. They said that the medicine would change her taste buds. Let me put it this way...she was given a Frosty—something that everyone loves—and, after taking three bites, said it tasted bad. *Tastes bad? Hmm. Let dear, old dad have a shot at it.* Seconds later, the taste test was concluded and the bottom of the cup had been attained. I would not say that it tasted bad.

The afternoon was spent in and out of sleep (more in than out). The nurses tell us that it's quite normal. Her stomach also began to turn, so she took some anti-nausea medicine to help. This of course has the side-effect of making her drowsy. Later, after giving it to her orally, we had one donning the rubber gloves and slipping her the puke bucket. Consequently she was soon off oral meds and slipped the 'ole IV injection. This is fine for the hospital staff, but what do we do when it's just us, back in the home away from home? And the rubber glove deal...well, that's because her vomit contains toxins which may irritate the skin.

Correct me if I'm wrong, but if I'm vomiting something that may irritate the skin, I'm thinking it must be some of the worst tasting vomit I've ever had pass through my mouth. Except for that one time as a kid I downed sour milk rather quickly one late night before realizing it had a funky taste. Sorry, didn't mean to go down that path and gross anybody out. On the upside, we are going to get a box of our own rubber gloves to take home! I'm sure the insurance company will cover it—hopefully (one box of toxin–proof rubber gloves, $150—not getting toxic vomit on you, priceless).

Tomorrow we get to check out.

Sharing the Experience

Today Hannah met a girl in the play room of the hospital. We had seen her before, playing quietly by herself as her dad looked on. Her hair is mostly gone, she seems confident in herself, yet she has a sense of need for support as her dad carries around the crutches she will eventually need. Back in March, she discovered that she has cancer in her leg.

Over the course of the day we had the opportunity to meet this girl and find out that she is in fourth grade, just like Hannah. As they talked a little, they tested the waters just as kids and adults do when meeting for the first time. Although as parents we jump right into conversation with others who are struggling with the how and the why of this disease. There are so many questions and so much to learn from those who have gone before you. It's hard to think that in a few short months we will be the ones talking to the "new" parents.

Cheyenne's dad told us how he came to find Mayo as a second home, and the Ronald McDonald House as a "getaway" from the hospital (they are a grand two blocks apart). Life as you know it stops. You take timeout of your everyday life to focus on the care of your child who now faces cancer.

I know Hannah had a zillion questions for Cheyenne, but when you're a kid, you simply want to enjoy the moment and the meeting of a new friend. Cheyenne and her dad will be here when we return. She is only a month and a half ahead of Hannah in her journey and is expecting surgery shortly. These two girls will have plenty of time to talk. So they spent time playing on the computer and enjoying board games today.

On a side note: I was taught how to give a shot today. Hannah has to receive injections for ten days following each treatment. I wonder if I could use this newfound skill as a classroom management technique—take your seat or receive a shot. No medicine, just the poke.

Released and Exhausted

Day 7:
Hannah had another long day of waiting. The chemo was complete, but the fluids needed to continue. About the biggest part of the day was the "dad shot." We decided to wait until later in the day to give the once–a–day shot because we have to give it around the

same time each day. Waiting for the shot is worse than actually getting a shot.

With a nurse looking over my shoulder, I completed the injection. Hannah rated me rather high on the scale of shot–ology. I tried to tell her that I had skills.

We went to visit the radiologist today as well. There was another set of doctors with another set of terminology and ways to handle the cancer. My favorite part is when they ask you, "Do you have any questions?" As if I could follow the jargon to begin with. Today we learned about "free radicals." You could tell the doctor wasn't used to dealing with kids. For all his efforts in explaining and drawing out how free radicals work and then further going into the chemical bonds of electrons and the DNA structure, his one question answered it all: "Now, Hannah, do you have an idea of what radiation is and will do?"

Hannah took no time in her response: "No."

And as any good professional would do, he quickly diverted the negative response to, "Well, maybe your parents can explain it to you later."

So ended our first radiology/oncology appointment.

This week we're back at the hotel awaiting more appointments. Take care for now and keep praying. The medicine is in her right now and hopefully destroying the tumor as we speak.

Tattoo, Wild Hair, and Drips

Day 8:

This was supposed to be a down day for us—short, sweet, and over by one o'clock. We were supposed to check in at the radiation therapy center, have them set up her radiation treatments, go get a wig, and go back to the hotel. Uh... not so fast.

Hannah had a rough night, which led into a rougher morning, followed by a "more rougher" afternoon. (I know that's not phrased correctly, I threw that in there for my students. Hopefully you picked up on the incorrect grammar and will let me know what the correct way to say it is.)

The idea of even keeping water in her stomach was beyond comprehension. The thought of food made her stomach turn. We were told that days following treatment might be full of nausea, but to actually go through it with her and to watch her energy drain from her body was very tough.

Yet, we had appointments, so off we went. Our first stop had us visiting the radiation center. The doctors kept telling Hannah that radiation didn't hurt and only lasted five to ten minutes. Not bad, right? They also told her that today was just a practice run to get the machines lined up correctly. What they failed to mention was the tattoo.

Tattoo? Yep, she would need to have a small dot made on her arm that would be a tattoo for the radiologists to follow as they moved her through the treatment.

"What does a tattoo involve?" was Hannah's question. It involved a needle, even I knew that much! Anything but a needle! Tell her she has to eat broccoli, but don't tell her she has to sit through another needle.

The resident doctor, who was explaining the procedure, not only tried to comfort Hannah, but agreed to get one first. The tattoo for radiation is a small dot on the forearm. They first placed a blot of ink on Hannah's arm, then the nurse took the largest needle I've ever seen (embellishment for reading pleasure), and she quickly poked it into her arm. With a wipe of the ink, the tattoo was in place.

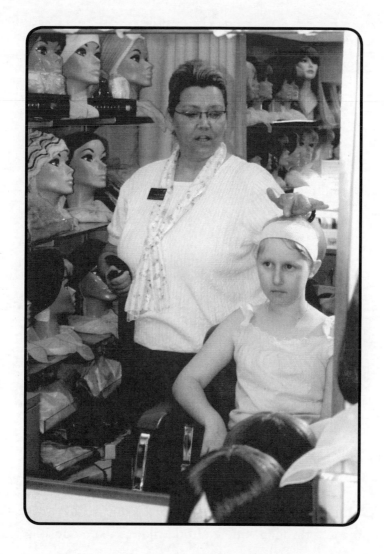

Our next stop on the trip was the wig shop. Following the first chemo treatment (approximately ten to fourteen days), your hair will begin to fall out in clumps. Most patients will seek a wig or wraps. We were even told that after a while, patients usually prefer one to the other. For now, Hannah was able to try on a number of hairpieces. They ranged in color and length. As she tried on a variety, she kept coming back to the third wig that she had tried. It looked an awful lot like her original hair. In between trying wigs, she was becoming weaker and sicker.

As wigs go, we found that most are worn in the wintertime—with a once in a while wear in the summer months (because of heat). Losing your hair is a tough thing. Knowing exactly when you're going to lose it is probably tougher. Not having been down that road, I can't speak for how hard it will be for Hannah.

After leaving the land of wigs, we made a path directly to the oncologist's office to have Hannah admitted for fluids and for some medicine to stop her vomiting. The doctors told us that in less than a day she had become dehydrated and lost five pounds. The importance of her drinking liquids and eating are crucial. Of course, it's easier said than done when you're not feeling well. Luckily she was in a place where we could see to her needs. A short day turned long, we made it through with a tattoo, wild hair, and one long drip.

There is a side note to our day. I can't believe I almost forgot. On our way out of oncology, we stopped to talk to a seventeen–year–old young lady who was in for her last visit. She had beaten cancer (a two year journey for her)! She gave us such hope and brought a smile to our faces. This is what this is about: telling your story, giving others hope, and showing that all things are possible. Luckily for us, she lives in Rochester, and we will touch base with her when we return.

On the Nines for a Blue Plastic Bin

Day 9:

It takes nine innings to complete a baseball game. It took me nine years from graduation to figure out what I wanted to be when I grew up. There are nine people in the Brady Bunch. I have nine toes (not really, but it works well with my story). It takes nine hours to get from Mayo to home. Coincidence? I think not—because we officially arrived back in Michigan on day nine!

Today began like the last, with a feeling of hope followed by a feeling of nausea. Of course, it waited to hit Hannah until we were actually at the Mayo Clinic, which I believe is approximately nine minutes from the hotel. We had three appointments to make it through today, and the first started something like this at the blood-drawing center (a favorite place for kids).

"Hannah Kelly?"

"She's here, but not present at the time. How do I say this ... she's vomiting at the moment." I spoke the words like a true guy–dad.

The blood drawing wasn't as bad as the carrying of the blue plastic bin through the hallways. Anybody who knows anything at Mayo knows that the blue plastic bin means: get to the other side of the hallway away from the person with the blue plastic bin. If you carry the blue plastic bin, you have a better chance of making it through crowded areas, having a private elevator, and getting to the front of the bathroom line. This is a *Saturday Night Live* skit waiting to happen.

We made our way back to the front entrance, discussing our situation the entire way. I believe it went something like:

"I knew she should have taken her anti–vomit medicine this morning."

"But she only needs it if she's feeling sick, which she wasn't."

"But who knows when it's going to hit you?"

"Exactly, so we need to get the medicine."

"But for the record, she should have taken it."

You see, as well prepared as we were with our paperwork, the medicine was going to take some getting used to. Hannah has about five various medicines to take, to help her with various symptoms of the chemo medicine. The one we needed at the moment was back at the hotel, of all the darned luck.

The quick thinkers that we were, we called the hotel and asked if they could scavenge the room and find the one white paper bag that held the miracle anti–vomiting medicine. A nine–minute trip later, and we were in business with that magical medicine.

Our next stop was the hand specialist, Doctor Alexander Shin. His job is to save the hand and as much function as possible following the surgery that won't be until later this summer. He laid out the three scenarios that he thought might be possible for Hannah's rebuild. Of course, he couldn't be sure which direction they would need to take until the tumor removal surgery had been performed. The first was that some function could be retained. The second was that a little function could be retained. The third was that no function could be retained, and the forearm would be lost.

I was able to take this all in with some degree of distance. Hannah, on the other hand, looked at us after the third option, gathered a little smile, and looked back at the doctor. She said, "What does that mean?" So, he told her.

And again she looked at us with such confidence that no matter the outcome she would be okay with it. Her unbelievable strength nearly brought me to the floor. How could a child of ten sit there and listen to the worst case scenario and be okay with it? I couldn't comprehend it at first. But then it hit me: she has faith beyond measure and knows that God has a plan. Her strength through this has become my strength.

Our last stop was the Oncology Department. It's just a formality to check Hannah's condition and send us home. As we sat in the waiting room, Cheyenne walked in with her dad and her two siblings (an older sister and a younger brother). She had two more check–ups this week before they could go home. Cheyenne will be back, though, for surgery in June. I told them we would see them soon. I knew we were in for the long haul over the summer and sharing this experience would be invaluable for all of us.

We received the okay from the doctor and headed out, excited to get back home to Michigan. After all, it was only going to be a nine–hour ride. It passes quickly when you know you're going to be back home among family and friends.

We have approximately twelve days before we have to return to Rochester for the summer. That's twenty–four hours multiplied by twelve. Is it a coincidence that it's divisible by nine? I don't think so.

This Side of Normal Feels Good

Day 10:
Ah, a day without a doctor visit. How nice it is to go through an entire day without going to one appointment, being poked, pinched, and generally stared at.

I realize it sounds as if I were the one going through it, but I must confess something. Maybe it's just me, or perhaps someone out there can admit to doing the same thing, but when the doctor has Hannah breathe in and out in those deep, deep breaths, I find myself taking those deep, deep breaths as well. I can't help it. I just find myself doing it and then looking at the doctor as if to say, "Don't you want to make sure my lungs are clear as well?" What's wrong with my deep, deep breaths? I usually get the stare but never get the satisfaction of one little listen. By the time the whole thing is done, I'm exhausted. I don't know if it's age or not, but breathing in and out (deeply) somehow makes me feel as if I just had a workout. If they had the Presidential Physical Fitness Award for the forty and over crowd, there would be a poster on the gym wall charting how many deep, deep breaths we would need to attain in a minute's time in order to qualify for the prestigious award. There would be that, and possibly shoe tying, since that's another area that seems to wind me.

Second confession: We didn't actually make it through the entire day free of medical stimulation. We were on the phone with the Oncology Department at Bronson Hospital (twice) and once with our very own pediatrician. No matter where we are, having doctor contact is a good thing. Tomorrow we meet with the oncologist in Kalamazoo to discuss a plan for if and/or when Hannah's ANC counts (white blood cells) drop below a level that they can fight off any virus. They also need to keep track of her blood counts more closely (more pokes—ouch).

You see, right now her bone marrow is not producing the white cells needed to sustain a healthy body. Hannah receives shots for ten days following her chemo treatment to help with that loss. The medicine she gets from her injections should help to keep her "counts" from dropping too low. You can get sick fairly easily and you really don't have a way to recover when you have low counts. At least that's the way it was explained to me. The oncologist at Mayo did tell us that over 50 percent end up back in the hospital for a couple of nights to receive fluids. We're banking on being the under 50 percent.

Batting under One Thousand

Day 11–12:
We spent yesterday traveling to the oncology department at Bronson Hospital in Kalamazoo. The doctors and nurses seemed very nice and very knowledgeable. We received another briefing on what cancer means, what to expect, what the medicine does, what the downfalls are, and so on. The doctor and the nurses probably thought we weren't paying attention, but the truth is, when you're traveling down this road, you have no choice but to pay attention. It was just the second time that we sat down with the three-ring binder full

of information. No matter how they explain it, the fact doesn't change that we are battling cancer and that there's no other way to go but forward. The protocol has already been determined by the doctors at Mayo, and our crash course in the medical field is well under way.

What we really wanted to know was Hannah's white blood cell count. The way it was explained to us is that if the count is over one thousand, it is good. When it goes below that number, you need to take precautions because germs can have their way with the body at that point. The purpose of Hannah's shots each day is to counter the low counts.

Hannah's counts came in around six hundred. *Oh no, that can't be good.* Out of the six hundred, the lab had to do a further count to tell us which of those are the fighters (fighting off sickness). A little while later, we received the news that around 250 were actually prepared for battle against any intruders in the body. I wish I had seen the movie *300* at this point—but I hadn't, so I had no reference to fall back on. I did see *Revenge of the Nerds*—a few taking on the majority.

Simply explained to us, Hannah needs to be in a clean environment as she goes into her low period. She also will become tired and want to rest more (sounds like my life). Today she has logged couch time and naptime, which is exactly what she needs to do.

Hannah also had a chance to visit her class earlier in the day. She received a quilt made by the Trinity Lutheran Quilters that was presented to her by her class. Little did the quilters know, but purple and pink are her favorite colors. I would have guessed "kelly green" myself.

Memorial weekend is one of cookouts, friends, and family. We are thankful to be home for it, but will have to pass on all the gatherings for now. Next year, though, we're planning on a big weekend!

You Go, I Go

Day 13:
Counts are still low—or so we think. We have to go and get a blood test tomorrow to know for sure. The question was do we stay in a safe, clean environment and hope germs don't get into her system, or do we venture out to the relatives' house where the large family is gathering for a Memorial Day feast of sorts? The doctors did say it was okay to be out and around people, just to stay away from the ones that you might see if you were...watching a zombie movie (those guys never look good).

Hannah has an Uncle Tim who loves to jump in with both feet when it comes to just about anything. When he heard that Hannah would be losing her hair, he didn't want her to go it alone, so he said she could shave his head. Of course, without his possibly knowing, it was going to be sooner rather than later.

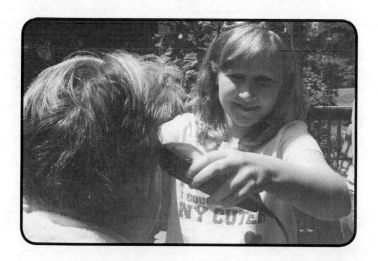

Good 'ole Uncle Tim has some thick hair that could challenge the sharpest of shears! However, that didn't make a bit of difference once the sound of the buzzers lofted through the air. We watched as Hannah maneuvered the clippers back and forth, taking the hair down like a combine at harvest time. You could tell she enjoyed herself greatly and appreciated the lengths at which her uncle had gone to be part of her experience.

With Hannah's chemo treatments, her hair will begin to go somewhere around the tenth to fourteenth day, but it could take as long as three weeks for the whole process. It's not quite as short as her uncle's process (which, I'm sure if you asked him, probably felt like a long time).

Backed by the Best

Day 14:

We can't begin to express our heartfelt appreciation for all the prayers, notes, posted comments, e–mails, phone calls, meals, assistance, and cards. Everyone deals with situations in different ways, but to know that we are not alone in our prayers is an awesome experience. No matter what wonderful physicians we have working on Hannah; it truly is a design of God.

Writing each day is a way to share our experiences, to reach out and communicate, and to ask for specific prayers. It gives us a feeling that although we're on the front line, we are backed by a strong group of prayer warriors.

We leave for Mayo on June 6 and don't expect to return until fall. Hannah has daily treatments of radiation scheduled, chemo every twenty–one days, and surgery set for the middle of August. From that point, we don't know what will be done. The doctors may keep us for further radiation and chemo, or they may send us home to have it done back in Michigan.

Hannah Has Her Say

Day 15:

From Hannah:

I just want everyone to know how much you mean to me. I think it's amazing that I have so many people praying for me. Since I've been going through so much, it makes me feel like they are going to take care of me in no time. Your prayers are going to help. I can feel the numbers of people praying for me, which makes me feel loved by everyone, my parents, and God.

I feel nervous about this summer and all the treatments. I think I'm going to be okay because God is with me.

I feel sad about leaving Saint Joe because I'll miss my friends and pets. I try not to think about my time spent in Rochester this summer. I just think about coming home.

Thanks for reading. I appreciate all the support and prayers.

Hannah

Hannah had another low day in the white blood cell count. She feels fine except for a rather raspy cough that occurs now and then. We hold our breath, waiting and praying and hoping that tomorrow brings an upturn to this slide in numbers. Of course, without our personal lab, we have no idea what the counts are doing. On Thursday she heads back to Bronson Hospital to find out the results.

Intentional prayers: Pray for the medicine to do its work on the tumor. Pray that her white cells rebound and that a healthy body is once again being produced.

Thanks for reading.

Sky–Rocketing Numbers

Day 17:

What a difference a day and a few hundred prayers make.

Hannah spent the better part of today at Bronson Hospital in Kalamazoo. As part of her weekly routine, her blood gets the once–over twice a week. When we last checked, her numbers had dropped rather low, and Kim and I were about to reenact *The Boy in the Plastic Bubble* (the movie with John Travolta) in order to keep her well.

Today her counts are not only up, but they have gone past normal straight to Superman status; or is it more appropriate to say Wonder Woman? The doctor gave Hannah the great news that the shots could stop, and she could go to school tomorrow. One of Hannah's biggest things this week was to finish out her school year with her friends. With tomorrow being the last day of school, the news and timing couldn't have been better. Prayers do work miracles.

The other side–effect to the chemo treatments is finally here—the loss of hair. As of yesterday, Hannah's hair began its commute south. It's strange in a way to look at her and see a clump of hair laying on her shoulders or shirt. You really can't tell where it's coming from ... it's just there. For most, I would think that this would be one of the hardest things to deal with. Well, unless you're Uncle Tim. In his case, he just got tougher looking.

Hannah and Kim are off to get her hair shortened a bit. She really does not want to go the route of bandannas, hats, or wigs just yet. As long as you can't tell that it's falling out and leaving large bald spots, she might as well keep as much as she can. I can understand that thinking.

We are planning on heading back to Mayo next week.

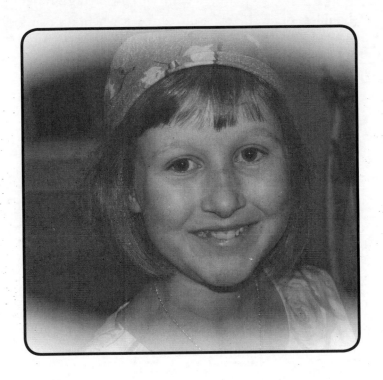

June

Spirit of Youth and God

Day 18:

After being out of the classroom for more than a month, going back for the first time can be a bit intimidating. Add to it that you'll have to sit in chapel with the entire school, and you may get the feeling that everyone is looking in your direction. Further this with the fact that your hair is beginning to just fall out in clumps, and you have to wear a bandanna, which is opposite from what others are wearing. Hannah, by personality, is not a person who likes a great deal of attention.

I suppose I could try and equate this to the time I got up in the morning, put on my clothes, and went to school. The problem wasn't my wardrobe of the day; the problem was that I had worn my pajamas under my clothes (I was six). I was certain that everyone knew. I looked like I gained twenty pounds with the bulging clothes, and I was completely devastated.

So how was it back at school? Throughout my day I kept wondering how Hannah was doing. I said a few prayers and had those feelings that a parent would have for his/her child who has to go through a difficult, awkward time.

After waiting for her to get home, I finally made the call home to do the questionable, "So, how was your day?" call. If you haven't seen a miracle before, it looks like this ...

Hannah not only went to school and had a great day (felt fine about the bandanna), but after school she went to a friend's house with a group of girls (without the bandanna). One of her friends had seen her without it on her head and told her that although she had some bald spots, she didn't look bad at all. That's all it took for her, and the bandanna was off for the rest of the day.

We pray for strength and for health (with her blood counts).

Fries with That?

Day 19:

With one last weekend to spend in Saint Joseph, along the shore of Lake Michigan, you tend to slow down and to notice things a bit more before moving out of your home for the next few months.

I've experienced being on vacation for a week, but this is like "snowbird" type stuff. I need retired–people help! Thank goodness we have parents: those who specialize in packing up, shutting down a house, and moving out for months at a time. If I were a betting person, I would say that retired people could possibly corner the market in this arena of temporary moves. Families across the nation would seek their help and advice. Heck, just getting mail taken care of seems like a PhD course.

Our plans are to stay at the Ronald McDonald House (RMH) for the summer. Being centrally located in Rochester, the RMH will provide us with the opportunity to be close to the Mayo Clinic and Saint Mary's Hospital. It's also just blocks away from downtown, tennis courts, and a McDonald's restaurant (for Max's Friday night Happy Meal fix).

The Ronald McDonald House has other opportunities available as well: a couple of grills, a small play area, a computer room, and a game room with the eighties game of all time: Ms. Pac Man and Galaxian in one glorious machine.

Hannah begins her second round of chemo this Friday—rev up those prayer chains. Following her chemo treatments we will be released from the hospital. Then she goes straight to her radiation treatments.

Last Day of School

Day 20:
This past week of school has gone by so slowly. With Hannah starting her chemo treatments today, I've been on my own in Michigan for the past couple of days. Sitting in my classroom today, with Kim, her mom, and the kids already off to Mayo, is like a slow drain on my emotions. Yet I have to put in my contract time, wrapping up final paperwork and packing things away in my classroom for summer cleaning. Honestly, knowing what I have ahead, taking care of the little things at school seemed pointless.

Tomorrow I hope to hit the road before the sun breaks the horizon. Too bad the forecast is calling for thunderstorms tomorrow because I'm riding the motorcycle to Minnesota.

June 7, 2007 (Day twenty)

From Kim's Journal:
We went swimming this morning, and what was left of Hannah's hair matted together. It was time, and she was ready. She asked me to cut it, and I did. It is not evenly cut, nor is it perfect, but in a way she looks

like Annie Lenox. She will be able to try all kinds of new hairstyles when her hair comes back in.

We went to see the radiation doctor. I like her and wish she was Hannah's doctor. She said we have a good plan—the main growth plates in her upper arm and wrist won't be touched by radiation. She said that years ago the only option with sarcomas was amputation. Now with radiation and chemotherapy there is a better outcome with how much the surgeon has to remove. She talked about internal radiation and more. She also reminded me that microscopic cancer cells can travel to the lungs. Instantly I find myself in that dark place—the one that scares me so badly that I can hardly breathe. So how do I stay positive when I go to that dark scary place ... the "what if I lose it" place? When I look at her with almost no hair, I feel sad— sad that she has to go through all of this and sad that she can't just do what other ten–year–olds do. I look at her, and my heart almost bursts with how much I love her. She troops through all of this so well.

Ah, Rochester

Day 26:
Back at Saint Mary's Hospital at the Mayo Clinic.
It's like we never left.
A home away from home.
A déjà vu.

A familiar feeling.

Been here, done it.

Amber, our nurse, picked up right where she left off with Hannah before we were dismissed after the first round of chemo—flush the body.

Hannah's first hook–up is not to medicine but to a saline bag that will saturate her body to prepare it for what's to come. Amber explained that once Hannah is sufficiently plump (with water), she would be ready to move forward.

How do they know when that happens? Easy, they measure the amount of liquid coming out. Once she reaches the equivalent amount, which could be enough to float a battleship, she's good to go. Think of it as a water balloon—the *perfect* water balloon. You want it to be just full enough to soak the intended target, yet not so full that it throws off your aim or pops on release.

So here we sit, waiting and becoming masters of the video–gaming world. The whole watering process will take about two hours.

Side note: I made the bike ride in ten hours (only fell asleep at the handlebars once). For those who don't have a motorcycle, it takes about $100 in gas to drive to Mayo. It took just over $50 by bike. Now, doesn't that make you want to run out and join a biker gang?

We are also in the Ronald McDonald House! By *in* of course I mean we threw everything in the room before heading to the hospital (a.k.a. the watering hole). We have yet to complete our entry briefing, so we aren't officially checked in. That's to say, the ladies running the place have a file folder with our name on it, and there's paperwork to be checked off. I hope they don't ask where I ate dinner tonight—KFC. It could mean an immediate expulsion.

Take Off and a Wedding

Day 27:

Breakfast arrives this morning followed by a child life counselor with the announcement, "Helicopter tour will begin in thirty minutes if you're interested." Did she say "interested"? Of course I'm interested. You may even go as far as to say, "enthusiastically interested." But, then I realized she wasn't talking to me.

One quick overview of the situation went something like this:

Hannah needs to eat her food. I need to run to the McDonald House for the camera and clothes, grab Max for the tour (because he's not only going to want to see the helicopter but fly it somewhere), and get to the family room at the hospital to meet everyone for the tour. That's not too much to do in thirty minutes.

The helicopter tour was sensational (and I'm not just saying that because I was the most fired up). Just being up on top of the roof and looking out over all of

Rochester and beyond was very cool! The flight nurse gave us the grand tour of the inner workings of a medical–copter. All in all, we spent some quality time up and out, which the doctors said was the best thing for Hannah.

Max found a new interest—for the moment. His biggest question was, "How close can we get to the edge of the building?" This was on the heels of the flight nurse's talk about being careful because they have no safety fence to catch you.

The wedding of the year is happening right now while we sit in a hospital in Minnesota. We are missing the union of Jen and Dave who start their new lives together as man and wife. I was supposed to walk Jen down the aisle and have the pleasure of giving her away, yet she understood why I would not be able to do so. This was an awesome responsibility (walking down the aisle) that I took seriously and practiced for hours, make that years. You could say I became a natural—at walking.

After realizing what we were into with Hannah, Jen graciously and lovingly said she knew I had to be with my family (even though she's a part of our family, and I think of her as my eldest daughter).

Since I couldn't be there for her on the big day, I just wanted to say these fatherly words: Have trust enough to know that God will direct your steps. Have strength enough to know that worldly issues should never interfere with your direction as a couple. Love carries you through the good times; love for God and family will get you through the rest. (There—that's my toast for my eldest.)

Intentional prayer: Pray for strength through this second round of chemo. Hannah made it through day twenty–nine, with her head tucked into her pillow for a long afternoon nap. We can see her energy level dropping.

Bubble Gum and Good Things

Day 30:
Today got off to a great start at ten a.m. (That's eleven for everyone back at home on E.S.T.). Hannah had been up through the night with bathroom trips, so sleeping in was a good thing.

Today treatments seem to be going similar to last time, which is another good thing because a surprise is not anything we need at this point. Hannah has become quite the wheelin'–about–the–floor–girl as she whirls her metal pole with fluids around like a date at a sock hop. Of course, her date is stiff with little action going on, other than an occasional beep. Just for reference, I do not know what a sock hop is...just what I've heard about. In my day, we were made to keep our shoes on at a dance.

The doctors stopped by this morning and gave us an update on her treatment schedule. They explained that after three treatments, they would take another MRI to see exactly what was happening inside her arm. That would be classified under "good thing" in the medical journals because we don't want them to just guess at it.

Amber, meet our friends and family. Friends and family, meet Amber, our nurse and resident bubble gum expert.

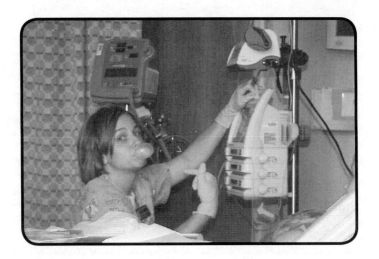

Amber and Hannah became chewing–gum girls today as Amber threw down the largest–bubble–in–the–universe contest. The photo above illustrates Amber's competence in backing what she says. Anyone wishing to challenge Amber need only to submit a photo to St. Mary's Mayo Eugenio Litta Children's Hospital, Rochester, MN. Amber would be more than happy to hear from you.

Amber is one of those special people that God places in your life just at the right moment. She was there during the motorcycle encounter, the helicopter happening, and through both treatments so far. Her personality and the way in which she interacts with children is truly a blessing for everyone under her care, which qualifies as a good to great thing. Not to mention that her husband rides a motorcycle, which puts them even higher in the *Book of Dave*.

We continue to ask for prayers and strength for Hannah as she enters her last day of treatment. Tomorrow we start radiation and recuperation at the Ronald McDonald House.

Watering Hannah

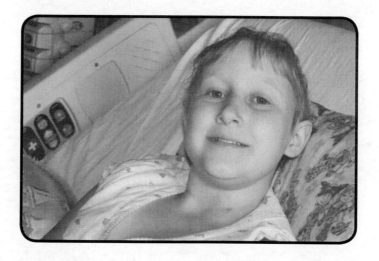

Day 31 (Part A):

Impeccable timing: the doctors walked in this morn-ing to give Hannah a check–up and to make a plan for today—when to release her, when to have her return for more fluids, how we could get a hold of them if things went downhill this afternoon. There had been a lot of *what ifs* as they talked amongst the group of doctors. As they were making the best possible plan, Hannah popped up in bed and began heaving into her bucket. Silence fell across the room as we all just stared at Hannah because there was nothing else we could do. When she had finished, red faced and drained, the doctors took the *what if plan* and said they would see us later today after her radiation treatment. We will not be going anywhere until late tonight.

The last day of chemo seems to also be the first day of nausea. Hannah's appetite goes and drinking water becomes the priority. We have a little game we play with the drinking part. It's simple: if we make eye con-tact, she has to drink.

For Hannah's part, she usually plays as if she's sleeping when I walk in the room (she's actually gotten quite good at it). I end up standing over her waiting for an eye to sneak open to see if I've gone, as a smirk comes across her face. "Ah, you're faking again! Now you owe me a drink!"

We're taking a different approach this time around with her medication. Last time we waited until she felt sick before trying to give her the anti–nausea meds, which technically speaking, didn't stay down. Now we're going to do the every–six–hour dose no matter what until she's through the first few days. She obviously feels better when her stomach is not spinning round and round, *like a record baby right round round round* (can you name that song?). The picture on page 69 is Hannah on her medication. I'll spare you the nausea pictures. (You're welcome.)

We pray daily that the chemo and the radiation are doing their prospective jobs by destroying the tumor.

What's a Transport?

Day 31 (Part B):
Between feeling sick and being hooked up to fluids, going to the radiation appointment was either going to be postponed a day (which would throw us off schedule) or the other option: "We've ordered a personal transport for you."

We thought a *personal transport* meant a personal taxi, instead of the shuttles that run all over Rochester. Imagine our surprise when two female emergency medical technicians from the Gold Cross Company showed up with a gurney.

Hannah later explained, "I thought it was really scary when they were pulling me up in the bed. I was just sitting there at a low level when they all of a sudden shot me up to their head height. The ambulance ride was kind of fun. They even ran the siren a few times so I could hear it. They couldn't run it too much because then people would begin pulling over. They were very nice."

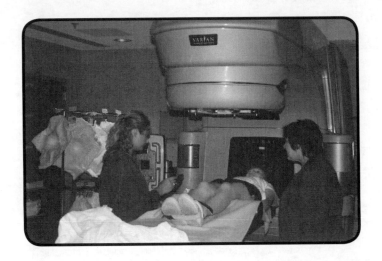

Hannah's radiation appointment went well, and we received another ambulance ride back to the hospital. When we returned to the room, we found a stuffed animal on her bed that was a gift from our new friends at Gold Cross.

By Grace and Mercy

Day 32:
Each day seems to hold a new eye–opening experience. Through God's grace and His mercy, we find

hope and belief that He has us in his heart and in his hands.

Today I met a family who has an eighteen–year–old son who is returning to Mayo with two tumors on his brain. When he was nine he had one tumor removed, and they felt that he was on the road to a normal, healthy life. They are back and live just down the hall from us at the Ronald McDonald House.

I also met a little girl who's ten. Her mother told us that she has Leukemia, and that her vertebrae are beginning to fuse together. She has to wear a brace around her mid–section to help her.

Another boy has tumors on both kidneys and a spot on his bladder. He was here to have his kidneys removed and was given medicine for his bladder. He has to live the next two months hooked up to machines to keep everything functioning. His dad said that once his son is strong enough, they are going to take one of his kidneys for his son, and then they'll both be in the hospital.

And then there's Cheyenne, the other ten–year–old girl we met earlier. She just finished surgery where a major part of bone was taken from her thigh and a bone in the lower part of her leg was removed and placed in her thigh. She lost a good amount of muscle during the surgery as well. She's stapled from hip to toe. The first day we saw her, she was so out of it that she couldn't remember really talking to me. Her recovery from surgery is expected to be about a month. Then she has rehab and more chemo beyond that.

There are many more stories that I could tell you, but I think you get the idea. You can't go far without sharing a story with another set of parents, seeing a child fighting through a disease that whose cause isn't understood, or meeting a family that is unsure that they will come out of this okay. Fear isn't around the corner—it's right in front of you. But you know the cool thing? Through faith we know that we have God standing in front of us, keeping the fear from reaching us. By his grace and mercy we are not alone.

One of the bright sides to this is the bonding and friendships that you make. Cheyenne's sister, Arianna, and Hannah enjoyed a good game in between all the medical action. For now, that's the best time in the world.

Peace and prayers.

"Search me, O God, and know my heart; test me and know my anxious thoughts."

Psalm 139:23 (NIV)

Too Much Time on My Hands

Day 33:
It's the second day out of the hospital, and all is well as long as we stay away from the research of Hannah's cancer. Just when we find time on our hands, the

Internet begins calling, and the research begins. I don't know why we look things up; it won't matter in the long run. I guess it's that we hope for positive information, something to give us that "whew" feeling. So, research it is.

In addition to a great deal of medical jargon, which I stumble through under my breath in order to not appear unintelligent, the articles seem to have a general theme—Hannah is a lotto ticket waiting to happen. Her type of cancer seems to be extremely rare in children, which makes the treatment fairly new. They have tested a number of treatments on adults, but children respond differently. So as they work on this pediatric cancer, it's all new to them.

We ask for your prayers that the tumor is being destroyed by the chemo and the radiation treatments. The doctors tell us that it won't be until July 26th when they perform another MRI and CT scan to see how the progress is going. Waiting is the hardest part. "*Deal or No Deal*" has nothing on this type of suspense.

Taking this journey day by day is the best medicine for us, along with a great deal of prayers. We are very thankful to have such a tremendous group of prayer supporters and caring people in our lives. It's wonderful and uplifting to receive letters and notes from you.

Hair Today, Town Tomorrow

Day 34:

It seems that the days just fly when you go from appointment to appointment. Of course, in between appointments we eat and relax. The nurse in radiation told Hannah that she may get tired, and when that happens, no matter when, it's okay to take a nap. This philosophy is right in line with my thinking! If I'm tired, a nap is in order. What adult wouldn't like that advice? Of course, I have to tell you in the only way Jody the Nurse could deliver it: "So, yay, okay, ya take dere nap when you feel tired, yay, okay den."

One of our appointments today was at the Wig Shoppe. Hannah received a new head of hair, Max was able to offer his opinion on just about every wig in the joint, and I got a new hat for tennis.

Strangely enough, though, Hannah had to get a haircut first. I kind of wish my hair went like this—the no fuss hair day where I would get up in the morning and put on my hair. There'd be no worries about washing or drying it, no combing, and no haircut ever required. Hannah's new hairdo looked great, and she gleamed with anticipation of going out on the town.

The daily shot and radiation treatment went well today. Hannah keeps count of her shots. It seems that Grandpa Kelly is going to owe her some cash when this is all over with. With the promise of a dollar a shot, he may want to get out the Help Wanted Ads.

Tomorrow it's more of the same, with blood work and a visit with the Oncology Department.

Another Successful Prayer Poke

Day 35:
Each morning begins with a shot for at least ten days after chemotherapy. The disappointing news for Hannah is that if she weighed over one hundred pounds, she would qualify for one adult shot and be done.

Each morning we head to St. Mary's Hospital for her fifth floor visit to the Infusion Center. I suppose if they called it the "Place of Sharp Needles" most kids would not get off the elevator.

Kim and Hannah start each poke with a prayer for strength and healing while they wait for the ice pack to numb her leg a bit more. Once the prayer is done, the nurse gets down to business.

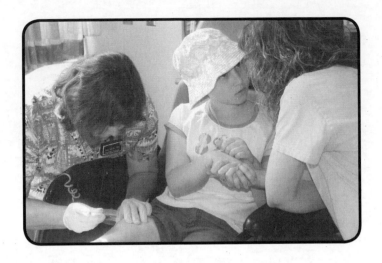

As the shot is administered, Kim and Hannah lock hands and eyes to begin the countdown. From zero to twenty, they count up. "One, two, three, four, five, six, seven, eight, nine, ten, eleven, twelve, thirteen..." A few louder numbers along the way usually indicates the burning that accompanies the medicine entering her leg. Once they hit the magic number, the needle is usually on its way out.

Heading back to the Ronald McDonald House is always more talkative than it is on the way to the hospital.

Another day of shots down; another prayer answered. Thanks, God!

Keep praying for Hannah's tumor destruction. Between the chemotherapy, the radiation, and your prayers, the tumor will be killed. We also ask for prayers regarding the tumor staying local.

Prayer and peace: they are truly uplifting.

Waiting Room Top Ten

Day 36:
"Is this what retirement feels like?" I solicited Kim's mom for future retirement information.

The days are filled with doctor visits and preparations for the next meal. In between these we manage a television show or video game. Yet, seven p.m. always seems to be just around the corner, and the day is coming to a close quickly.

"This is exactly what it's like—fast," was her response.

When we're not in the hospital, we're running to the hospital for infusions. When we're not running to the hospital, we're running downtown to the clinic for checkups. When we're not running for checkups, we're running for radiation. When we're not running for radiation, we're doing blood work. When we're not running to blood work, I come up with things to write about.

Here are my top ten things to do while sitting in a waiting room ... umm, waiting.

10. Play "Guess the Patient." When a group of people walk into the waiting room, try and guess which one is the patient.

9. When the nurse comes out to call the next patient, always start to get up as if it's you. (Start to stand.) "Oh ... that's not me." (Sit back down.) Repeat the process over and over and over again.

8. Grab a stack of magazines and try to read through each one looking for your name. Whoever has his or her name appear the most, wins. Also, the person who has the most magazines is loathed by everyone else in the waiting room.

7. Clip your toenails. (We haven't done this one yet, but I may get pushed to the brink of trying it).

6. Have a fashion contest—only don't let the rest of the patients know they're in the contest.

5. Bring a good book, but be ready to read the same page over and over again because the ladies sitting behind you are sharing their afflictions with one another in a manner that you can't help but listen.

4. Bring some dice, find some youngsters, and make some money!

3. Vator race! You have time; they have elevators. Race to the top, back to the ground floor, and back to your waiting room area.

2. The Aunt Joyce game. Try and get to know everyone in the entire waiting room area before being called.

And the number one thing to do while sitting in a waiting room is:

1. Act like it's *The Price Is Right* when you're finally called (even though you know you're just going to the back to sit in a small room for another fifteen to thirty minutes).

Today's blood transfusion went well (long, but well). With Hannah's blood results, we needed to head in this morning to boost her hemoglobins. With radiation, the oncologist likes to see her numbers higher than what they were. The transfusion was a total of just over a pop can's worth, but they have to do it slowly, so it takes hours to complete.

The remainder of the day was spent lying low.

When in Rome

Day 39:
The Loss of Hair, By Hannah:
It all starts when you have chemo from having a tumor. First, your hair just falls from your head, and it doesn't hurt. Some people are amazed at how you can just take your fingers and go through your hair, and it comes out. Cool, isn't it?

When a lot of hair starts to fall out, you have to finally go get it cut because your mom is tired of having to pull it off your PJs. So you're off to the hairdresser. The first thing they ask is, "Would you like to wash your hair?" I didn't want to, but I had to, so she did. Big surprise, my hair went into a big ball. I ended up with a chunk coming out and a big bald spot on the back of my head. She finished cutting my hair, and we left.

I could feel the bald spot. When we got into the car, I started to cry, and so did my mom. It was horrible. We went home and cried some more. After a while of crying, though, we got over it, and I got used to my shorter hair.

When we arrived in Rochester with my mom, Max, and Grandma for my second round of chemo, we stayed at a hotel with a pool. Swimming pool–cool! We went swimming and more hair bunched up–not cool. My mom ended up cutting it shorter until no more hair fell. I now have short, short hair. You end up used to it.

We have been enjoying "Rochesterfest" somewhat (it's a two week long festival). The other day we made it out to the dog and Frisbee contest and to visit the local population of Canada geese. They have a number of activities each day, but with Hannah approaching her lowest blood counts, we're taking precautions by limiting our outside House involvement. Hopefully by the weekend counts will be up in time to make the parade, balloon launch, and even the plane pull. You betcha!

Tied to the Calendar

Day 40:
The infamous "Desk R"—R for radiation, of course.

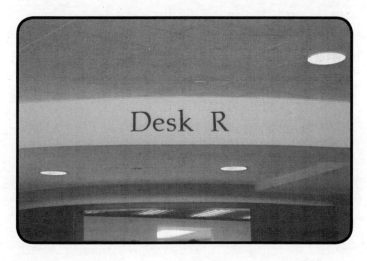

The empty calendar—is there such a thing? I'm thinking *yes*, but you have to be that guy on cable who gets dropped in the middle of nowhere. (I believe he's Survivor Man or something of that nature). He doesn't seem to have a calendar, but he does have an agenda.

We seem to start off the week with one, maybe two, appointments scheduled per day. Yet, *don'tchaknow*, each day brings a set of new appointments. We make one call to check on a current appointment and find that we've been scheduled for more. It's another good reason we're right here at the clinic, but some of these appointments seem … well, ap*point–less*.

For instance, Hannah met with a nurse today and discussed whether she preferred coloring or dolls. *What?* Of course, they disguised the search for play-time information by asking the all–important billing question: "Do you have any questions of us at this point?"

That last question she asked is the ultimate of questions. I, in typical fashion, like to ask them a question in return (like a matching of wits as it were, a mental volley back to their court). I usually like to throw out the double reverse question of, "What would be a good question to have answered at this point?" They typically, in solid form, shoot back with a statement of, "That's a good question," followed by a stare and long pause. Oh, you could cut the tension of the match with a plastic knife. We concluded the all–important meeting and moved on. I told Hannah that the nurse was more than likely looking for Christmas ideas for her own daughter or granddaughter.

They had animals on the loose today as they celebrated the opening of the sixteenth floor as the new all inclusive pediatric floor of the Mayo Clinic. The place was crawling with animals from the Minnesota Zoo as well as those in fuzzy, two–legged costumes. The new floor will host all pediatric patients. Currently, kids are spread out among the various departments on a multitude of floors. If you need blood–work you go to the subway level; for pediatric oncology you would go to a different floor. This new design of putting everyone on one floor will allow pediatric medical staff to work more closely together. The whole floor will actually open in July. The good news is that we'll be here for it. The bad news is that we'll be here for it.

We did get the blood counts, and her white cells are low, as we expected. The nurse recommended keeping her away from anyone sick. So everyone who's sick out there, cancel your plans of dropping everything and flying out here for the next day or two.

Hannah is in great spirits that her counts will be up very soon and that Buffalo Wild Wings are just a day away! It's our getaway time when we can go grab some wings. It's as if the chemo medicine isn't bad enough on her system, we go in search of something more!

I'll be sure to shoot some pictures of the balloons. Someone might need to give me a ring to get me out of bed, though, because it's starting at six something in the "Oh My Gosh It's Morning" time.

Rainy Dog Days

Day 42:
Today began like it left off yesterday—rainy. With forty–two rooms in the Ronald McDonald House with an average of two kids per room, that means eighty–four kids looking for inside action. You either plan something to do or find the nearest bottle of Tylenol. We had appointments to go to, as always.

The blood test didn't go so well this morning as Hannah's nurse had to access her twice because the first port access did not seat well the first time in order to get a good blood draw. "Grandpa owes me two dollars," is what I heard from her as she exited the blood center. Apparently, she's getting used to the port access part of life.

Once we finished with the blood work, we were off to the radiation for a quick once over and a chat with the doctor. Each week the doctors like to sit down and evaluate how the treatments are progressing. "Why are we just sitting here?" Sam questions while waiting in the waiting room for the first time. I smiled at him all the while thinking, *poor guy never read my "Top*

Ten Things to Do in a Waiting Room." I also gave him the fatherly reply of, "Because we're family, and this is what we're doing...all summer," as I plugged my iPod in and cranked up the volume just enough to make him wonder what I was listening to. He had forgotten his iPod back at the room. Life lesson learned: come prepared.

The blood work returned today with counts very high! The only low issue was the platelets (those are the things that keep you from bleeding excessively). So for now, we'll un–enroll Hannah in that bungee course.

The afternoon was spent having a visit from a dog named Kaja (Take your best guess at the pronunciation. I have no idea). The kids really loved hearing what the work dog did and loved petting him even more.

Following the visit from Kaja, the kids were treated to the craft of tie–dye! Most people pick clothing (T–shirts) to tie–dye, but our house child–life specialist, Kim, had the kids using pillow cases. How cool is that! Had I known they were doing pillowcases, I would have been up for joining them.

Thanks for all your prayers. Hannah is responding to her treatments very well (by no accident—that's prayer at work). We also ask that you continue to pray for the chemo and radiation at work in her. Pray that it is doing the job on this cancer.

Third is Number One

Day 44:

With the weekend coming to a close, we are looking at a week of radiation, but no shots!

The third week is always the best week (in a bittersweet way). It's the week that shots are done, counts are up, and feeling healthy and active is at its peak. It's also the week that as it comes to an end, another round of chemotherapy begins, and the process starts all over.

This past week has been fantastic when it comes to "things to keep us busy." With the Rochesterfest in full swing, there were a number of activities to go to, including: the balloon race (yes, we all made it there and then went right back to bed), the 1860s baseball game, and the flags of the 173rd Airborne lining an entire football field adjacent to Soldiers Field Veterans Memorial.

The other wonderful activity was the visit from the Simpson family. They drove to Minnesota for the weekend. It's always a good dose of medicine when you can spend time with friends. Just visiting and talking with friends is always a bit of home.

The hardest part of saying goodbye is not just saying goodbye to friends you won't see for months (or longer), but it's the fact that they get to go back home and continue on. Our journey, our life, is here, and although we have the great support of many, it's still something we can never just walk away from. I suppose that's what makes a visit from friends so special and why it's so hard to say goodbye. Friends and family can give you that relief from the here and now, from the situation you've been forced to deal with. Friends and family can make you have that feeling of…well, normalcy.

We thank God for our loving friends and family that give us such boundless comfort.

Quick Honk Chemo

Day 45:
I can't believe I just typed "Day 45" as if we just began this whole thing not long ago. I can't really say *time flies when you're having fun,* but I suppose I can say it has gone faster than I would have thought.

This Friday we ready ourselves for another long weekend at the hospital as Hannah enters her third round of chemotherapy treatments. This one will be without one of the big-dog medicines because of the way it interacts with the radiation. So, of course, we thought we would cut our time in half in the hospital and only have to stay a day and a half. No such luck.

We typically check in Friday (late morning/early afternoon) and start the fluids for the first dose. With Hannah's response to the medicine so far, we're hoping to stay the course and not run into any problems. She still maintains a shallow margin of hair on her head (all around). I believe she thinks she'll go the distance without losing anymore.

Hannah's finding out a bit of what daily writing is like since we gave out her e-mail. This morning she sat at the computer for about an hour trying to respond to most of the e-mails. She still has some to go. She said, "I love writing to my friends. It makes me feel as if I were kind of with them."

Tomorrow we're off to a baseball game (the Honkers) with a group of about thirty people from the House. The more to keep us busy, the better! Take care, and keep praying.

Peace and prayers.

Through You

Day 46:
Rather than write about us, I wanted to share with you what others have written to us through e-mails and comments left on the blog. Your words reach us with such power and with such faith that when I go to say my prayers, I know that there are hundreds of others kneeling next to me.

"Your extended family holds all of you in our prayers!"

"Yesterday will always be history, and tomorrow will always be a mystery, but today is the day to live for!"

"Three girls (age nine to eleven) made a special prayer quilt from fabric collected from their own baby clothes. The main purpose is for these girls to share with Hannah that they care, and they are praying."

"There are no words that can be written or said for the place you are. Take a deep breath, give yourself a big hug, and know the prayers are there."

"I pray that God will give Hannah the strength to endure the treatments. I pray for Kim and Dave the patience and contentment to lean on God for all that you need."

These are just a few of the words we receive daily that build our strength and rejuvenate our spirits. Thank you for your kindness, your love, and above all, your faith that God has a plan, reminding us that sometimes we must be still and listen.

Thank you. Peace and prayers.

Twenty Questions and Then Some

Day 49:

We had a terrific end to our week: grandparents arrived, we ate wings (the other method of chemo), and we went to the Mall of America. What is it? When I can walk around work all day long I'm fine, but for some reason you put me in a mall, and I'm good for about an hour before I'm suddenly tired. My feet hurt and my legs develop pains that only an Olympic runner might experience while training in a desolate wasteland. The whole experience of shopping is to see if I can walk from the bench I'm currently sitting on to the next bench twenty yards down. Oh yeah, don't forget the positioning factor because there are other guys in the mall doing and experiencing the same thing (so they, too, want your bench).

We're back in St. Mary's Hospital and beginning our third round. Here's the test to see if you're a novice or a veteran patient: how many questions can you ask? As a novice you really don't know what to ask, so you usually just stare a lot. As a veteran, it's attack and don't look back.

We had a *new* nurse checking us in and administering the needle to the port. By new I mean one we hadn't seen before. He introduced himself and rather than going through the cordial sequence, it was an immediate, "How long have been working here?" "Almost a year and a half," was the reply.

You could see Hannah giving it some thought. "How many ports have you accessed?" she questioned as the pokee.

"Not a great deal, but the ones I have done have been successful." Long pause. "Would you like me to have an expert do it?" he questioned further.

More awkward silence.

"What's not many?" Hannah continued the questioning for quite some time. She was not about to go through a novice–needle nurse just to make him feel better. He finally suggested having another nurse present, who had plenty of experience, and could assist if needed.

The port access went very well, and the nurse can now chalk up one more on the experience chart. Of course, we haven't had one nurse yet that wasn't top notch.

We did learn this week that Hannah's radiation treatments will end in the next two weeks. The doctors will be reviewing her case and will make recommendations from that point. We were told that her protocol is more of an outline of what should be done in terms of radiation and chemotherapy treatment. It's a flexible plan that doctors can change on a patient basis.

We also learned the word *hemoc*. Apparently Hannah falls into the category of a "hemoc child." Hemoc is short for combining hematology and oncology. I'm thinking of a shirt design. All others are allowed to participate by sending suggestions, drawings, sketches, and ideas—just mark it as "shirt me."

Intentional prayers: that Hannah has a good third round of chemo and that the medicine continues to breakdown the cancer cells.

This is Why We Pray

Day 50:

When you have time on your hands and you're in the hospital, you have a few options...Wimbledon is number one (but I'm just the dad). Then there's the Westminster Kennel Club Best in Show Competition. It went quickly from Best in Show to a Best New Friend for Mojo. After all, how could I resist getting another cute dog when they all look cool? Of course, those who know me know that Mojo is enough. Kim and Hannah even combined to give me the mother–daughter smile to try and soften me.

For those who don't know the name, Mojo is our American bulldog that is large enough to make up two dogs. After today's show, Hannah and Kim both began burning up the Internet looking at dogs/puppies. This is your chance everyone, aside from the hemoc "shirt me" contest (see day forty–nine), to throw in your two cents on your favorite breed (either as a friend or chew toy for Mojo).

Day fifty went by slowly with naps thrown in here and there. With the ups and downs of the previous night, we found it not uncommon to have Hannah nap a little off and on throughout the day. Josh was back on the job today as Hannah's nurse. He came in to check Hannah's vital signs and instantly became engaged in our puppy discussion, along with the Westminster Kennel Club Best in Show frenzy of the "oh they're so cute looking" hour. Josh returned later in the day and was kind enough to print out some possible pups for us. *I didn't even know a puppy was something on the table for discussion.* The Great Dane was among his favorites. Let's remember people, I live in a small house.

Hannah is doing well (with only a slight dip in her phosphates) after her first set of chemo drugs. Josh ended up pumping in some medicines to help with that. She begins her second round tonight with something called Mesna—a medicine that helps protect the bladder from the chemo. It begins working, and then comes the chemo medicine.

This time around Hannah only receives one of the two meds she had been taking. With radiation, the Doxorubicin can't be given in combination with it because it will severely burn her from the inside out. We thought it might be a shorter stay in the hospital, but we were wrong. The Ifosfamide is a three dose, three night event.

I know a great number of prayers are being said, but I thought I would give you a visual of what the tumor looks like:

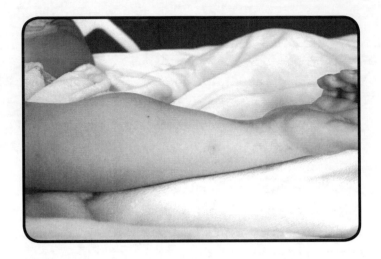

The tumor is closer to her elbow than the wrist. The tiny little black dot is the tattoo radiology gave her to assist in lining up the machines.

If you're searching for a few words in prayer, I tend to go with my standard:

Dear God: Kill this thing! Thanks.

July

What I Know or Not

Day 51:

I know that I'll never be a Pussy Cat Doll. I know that the Ronald McDonald House does not serve fries. I also know that for the better part of today, my watch read thirty–one on the date (but in my mind I kept telling myself it was actually the first and that I would have to find some way to change it—eventually).

Despite my wealth of knowledge, these are not the things that most people keep writing or asking about when they say, "What do you know?"

Hannah has about two more weeks of radiation, followed with one more round of chemotherapy sched-uled in twenty–one days. After that, we're scheduled for a set of scans that will give us more information. The doctors will determine at that point whether more chemo and radiation are needed, or if we proceed with the surgery which is currently slated for August 14.

Here's what I don't know ... if they will actually do a scan prior to July 26. One of our oncology doctors had mentioned *possibly* having a scan sooner. I don't know if radiation will end on the sixteenth because the protocol we're following has Hannah receiving radiation right up to her fourth round of chemotherapy. It seems that cancer is pretty much a try and check process. The problem with this is that we would like the check to happen quicker. I do know that the chemo takes time to work, so the checks will have to wait.

We got outside for a brief moment this afternoon. You have to love the warm summer breeze that just wraps itself around you. Now all we're missing is a sunset over Lake Michigan.

Peace and prayers.

Get Up, Get Out

Day 52:
Monday, 1:05 p.m. (that's 2:05 for those on EST): It's been widely agreed upon (during a phone conversation) between Van, my good friend from back home, and myself that central time is where it's at! You get to catch prime time starting at seven, news by ten, and to sleep by eleven. The bonus: when you wake up at

seven, you know that it's really eight and you just got an extra hour. It's like switching with DST everyday.

The goal for today is to get healthy quick. Hannah is desperate to be de-accessed (that's where they pull the big needle from her port) and get out of here. In order to do that, she needs to eat and drink on her own and keep it down. We have radiation by three, so she has two hours to get it together.

"I feel perfectly fine. I don't feel sick, but I don't want to eat anything from the kitchen," declares Hannah in her best persuasive voice. Too bad it's not working for Kim. She's insisting on food. Moments later they agree on splitting a salad. "While you're gone, can I pack my bag?" Hannah probes to hear the confirmation that she's one step closer to getting out of the hospital.

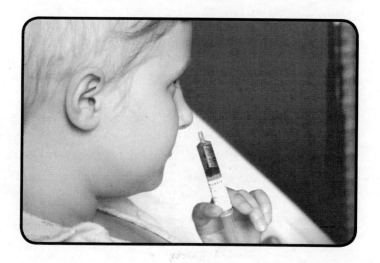

One of the other steps to getting out of the hospital is downing all the oral meds. With each tube that rolls in the door, Hannah has to give it the sniff test. It's become a standard for her. I'm not really sure if she can actually smell anything.

"Can you smell the medicine when you sniff it?" I questioned her.

"Sure can," she confidently replies.

"And?" I waited for her to add a bit more. It reminded me of being back in the classroom teaching.

"It's hard to say." She quickly flips the TV to another *Hannah Montana* show and blocks any more incoming questions.

So, there you have it. A definite "maybe it smells, maybe it doesn't smell like anything, but it is worth taking the time to give it a sniff."

Fire Up the Grill

Day 53:

No matter what we have going on, the smell of a grill is just one of those smells that always brings the olfactory senses around to happy memories.

We've kind of made a tradition of firing up the grill whenever Hannah gets through another round of chemo. So the next time you're out stoking the coals or turning up the heat on that gas grill, take a deep, deep

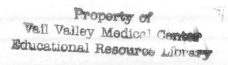

breath and think of us in Minnesota as we think of you back home and around the country.

Hannah finished her fiftieth shot this morning. As we were getting ready to head to the hospital, the anxiety began to build. I guess it doesn't matter if it's the first or fiftieth shot. None are easy to prepare for.

As we prepared for the injection, the nurse gave the "Are you ready?" cue, and Hannah took the deep breath, looked at Kim, and said, "Not now, in just a minute."

The shot went off well, with her and Kim's count only topping fourteen, and it was all over. Next stop radiation.

Hannah's getting to be regular at the radiation desk as she nears her fifteen out of twenty–five treatments. I asked if it's possible for me to travel to the back room with her and get some photos. She thinks it won't be a problem, but she needs to clear it first.

Tonight we went to our first support meeting for parents whose children have cancer. I must say I'm not much of a meeting guy. I envisioned the grand greeting of "Hi, Dave!" followed by some form of group hug, but as usual, I was wrong.

The Brighter Tomorrows group was started by parents who have been through what we are experiencing. No medical staff can say, "Go down the hall, and you'll find parents who are experiencing things you're going through" (confidentiality issues). Yet parents can seek out others—you just look for the bald kids. You know that the kids are looking for others just like them, and the parents are looking for other child cancer parents. We were also clued in that at the hospital, the hemoc kids have trains on the door by their room number so you can go down the hall and check out tags for trains.

Tonight's topic was on building photo memories and journaling. Check. I had been taking photos, writing about our experiences, and making DVDs along the way. It was good to be on top of something for a change. With cancer, you never know where you stand, what's going to happen the next day, or if what you're doing is the right thing. At least with journaling and the photos I could sit back and comfortably say, "Everything is under control." That's the hardest part of this cancer journey … turning it over. Yet when you can step back and look at the big picture, there's really nothing else you can do.

Fireworks and the Queen

Day 54:
It's day fifty–four, but I didn't have the stamina to write on day fifty–three (with the fireworks followed by a late family movie back at the Ronald McDonald House). It wasn't our traditional cookout like back in Saint Joseph where we have an open invitation for

everyone. The cookout is followed by a walk to the beach on Lake Michigan for fireworks, then back to our house where we reopen all the leftover food from earlier. This year we were up late and overloaded with food as usual, but the two items missing were friends and Lake Michigan.

Ah, fireworks over Dairy Queen. You have fireworks at Disney World, fireworks over Lake Michigan, and then running a close third are the fireworks over Silver Lake (or as close to Silver Lake as you could get with the large crowds encircling the small lake) in Rochester.

Not being familiar with the protocol of a new city—where to park, where to go, where the best seats are, when to leave to avoid the traffic, we opted for the "close enough" venue. So we headed for ice cream and decided to stay at the DQ for the show. We knew it was a good decision when Max screamed out among the other DQ patrons, "These are the best seats ever!" Sure they were. You have fireworks, ice cream, and extra chocolate all right there.

Hannah loved being out right up until the mosquito bite. You think about mosquitoes, but you never react to them like you do when you have a child with no—or little—hair. Now that I think about it, we reacted the same way when the kids were newborns: protect them at all cost from the mosquitoes! You get out the big, tropical rainforest netting and blanket them with it.

Unfortunately, our netting was being dry–cleaned, so we did the next best thing—took some pictures, got the last *oohs* and *aahs* in, and headed for the car. With each turn down a new road, we had to adjust the kid's sight to see the fireworks. "Look out the left window, now the back window, right between the trees, now the left window again." Amazingly enough, back at our room we had a perfect view of the firework finale over Rochester.

More Than a Day

Day 55:

It's been a busy end of the week for us. Grandma and Grandpa Kelly left for home, Sam and I got in a motor-cycle ride to the Mighty Mississippi, we were adopted by a very cool family, and we moved up in rooms. The House has a variety of rooms, and we began with one of the smaller ones (I mentioned the name of George Jefferson, but it went completely over Sam's head).

We said goodbye for now (which is more like, "see you very soon") to Grandpa and Grandma Kelly as they headed back to Hoosier Land. Sam and I had the opportunity to get out for a ride, so we gave them an escort as far as the turn off to Winona. We headed north toward the bend of Mississippi as they went east to LaCrosse. There's something about getting out and riding the hills of Mississippi. Of course, we could spot Grandma behind us with her camera at the ready.

I can't believe I almost forgot to mention that James and Christine had a baby boy. Evan is brand new to this family thing as James and Christine figure out what to do with their first child. This is where Kim and I were supposed to swoop in and help them; having three kids makes you a semi–expert in the field. Unfortunately, they will just have to manage for a while without us, until we return.

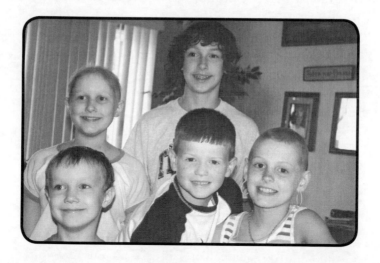

Later in the day, we had the opportunity to spend some time with a family who has already been down the road we are traveling. Their daughter, Danielle (who's eleven), was diagnosed with cancer around April 2006. Danielle finished her treatments this past spring and is doing great. Being in the area, they have become a great comfort and resource for our family.

They have asked us if it's okay if they adopt our family. Talk about a choked up moment. It was one of those times that I couldn't really speak because I was so overwhelmed that people whom we had just met not only invited us over to their house for dinner, but also wanted to help us through this rough time. It's a huge pay–it–forward moment and an answer to prayer once again. We ask for strength, and God gives us a family that has been down our road, right here in Rochester. With their son, Collin (who's six), it's been a great match for the kids. Did I mention that Steve is a coach (women's basketball at the local college)? Darn all the luck that we'll have to talk ball. We might even get some court time with Hannah if she's up to it. Coaches always have keys to a few gyms.

The last monumental thing to happen at the end of this week—other than having Max turn from a six–year–old to a seven–year–old—we had the chance to move up to a bigger room. It's not one of the bigger rooms that we were hoping for with *two* rooms. Yet, it's about fifty square feet larger than our previous. And with five people sharing one room, we'll take it! Sam was so excited that he took on the role of "One Guy and a Cart." He was hauling rubber bins as fast as we could fill them.

Last but not least (which means you'll probably hear more about it). Under the good intentions of keeping busy, the family held a family vote, which has resulted in enrolling me into a tennis tournament. They have vowed to provide Advil, rubs, and other comforts to ease my pain when it's all over, so I had no choice. I believe the words that broke me were, "Come on, Dad, just do it!"

Well, heck, who can say no to that logic? It's a NW sectional for Minnesota (which means I'm way over my head). The bonus: because I signed up today, I get the pleasure of starting with a seeded player. Bets can be made now on how long I last on the court (in minutes, not hours). Closest to the total time as well as a win/loss will receive a gift. You have one week to submit. Tournament begins Saturday.

Peace and prayers.

Oh—you wanted to know about Hannah? How could I forget her? Her counts are up at the moment, with another check on Tuesday (which they should be a bit lower). She is doing great according to her doctors. We have six more radiation treatments to go! Prayers are a powerful thing, along with faith (and she's a testament to that).

Re-energizing

Day 57:

It's one of those nights where my body says, "call it a day," but my mind has about twenty thousand things going through it, and they are all taking turns rattling around in my head. So what's the solution? You jot stuff down.

Our "adoptive family" (this is the official point at which I will stop calling them that) left for the weekend, but they left us with a key to their home and an open invitation to use their house as our own. Heck, I have trouble letting someone in the front door of my house when there are shoes scattered all over, the sink is full of dishes, and backpacks are blocking the back porch. The Huckes, who are just getting to know our family, turned over their entire house (and their four wheelers for the kids). This family is amazing and a Godsend.

We spent about four hours there today, swimming, grilling, and you betcha... riding the four wheelers. It was a tremendous getaway that we not only needed but thoroughly enjoyed. As I sat out on the deck reading from a Coach K book and listening to the sizzle of brats as the juice made the flames climb higher, I couldn't help but think, we need to re-energize as often as possible.

There are so many turns in our day where we can have the energy zapped out of us without even realizing it. Yet there are just as many, if not more, things in our day that bring a smile to our faces. Getting mail (both regular and electronic) is one. Talking on the phone with friends, receiving pictures, hearing about the prayer groups and the kind actions of others, making new friends, and so many more things all re–energize us.

I guess as I sit alone in the day room, late, late at night, I can't help but to want to call each and everyone of you *right now* and say, "Thanks for re–energizing us, now go back to sleep." I'll spare you the phone call, since it is the middle of the night. You're welcome.

Oh, and Van, if you're reading this, for all the times you woke me early on my day off or on a lazy Saturday morning, just know you would have been the first call!

A Walk in the Park

Day 59:

Monday morning and we're back on schedule with our daily routine of infusion and radiation. We typically begin the morning by pumping loads of caffeine into our bodies (Kim and I that is) while the kids begin another morning of "let's see what's on channels sixty through sixty–nine" (the kid stations). After a brief thirty minutes of looking over the daily schedule, we head down to the kitchen for breakfast. We share our kitchen and dining table with roughly twenty other families, so it makes for a Golden Corral experience at times.

Hannah has been handling the shots better, but I suppose if you were to ask her about them, the words *I hate them* and *shots hurt* would be among the general description. She still gets out every morning to head off to the infusion center at the hospital, where one of her favorite injectors (that's code for *nurse*), Donna, gives her the shot. Donna has a nice touch, as many of the nurses do, but for some reason she has successfully achieved the "*great shot giver of all time*" award for Hannah.

Typically we head off to radiation by mid–morning. Hannah gave me the okay to follow her back down the long hallway to the radiation room where she gets set up for her daily dose of radiation.

The whole room, including the rather large machine under which she lays, is a little intimidating. However, when you go through something every day, it becomes a walk in the park. Hannah had no sign of intimidation as she hopped up on the table to ready herself. The nurses take a form and place her arm in it just so, and then laser lights shoot beams on all over the room. You can't see them in the photos because my flash kept washing them out, but trust me on this one, they are all over.

One of the coolest parts (if there truly is something cool to your child receiving radiation) was when a lighted measuring tape appeared on her arm and one nurse called out the number for the day. The nurse then began moving the machine until the laser lined up with the measurement. See, another reason to pay attention to measurements in school. She would pass my class. She is smarter than a fifth grader!

The last step is literally taking one step backward (for those of us with two feet still on the ground at this point). The machine moves in closer to Hannah as we get out of the way. In fact, I think their exact words were, "Hey, Dad, move it!" They take one last look, pop in an audio CD of Hannah's choosing (even doing track requests) before having everyone exit the room.

The nurses then operate the radiation machine from their command center across the hall. They get to watch the whole thing through satellite imagery (or closed circuit television, which doesn't sound as exciting). I thought for a moment that I might be able to observe the whole process—until one of the nice nurses gave me directions back to the waiting area. I can take a hint on most days. Good thing this was one of them because I wouldn't want to embarrass my ten-year-old. For some reason, that phrase keeps coming up a lot: "Dad, don't embarrass me." They haven't seen me play competitive tennis yet! Anyway, another day of radiation, another day at Mayo.

We give thanks for everyone reading, praying, and supporting our family.

Living Ronald's Way

Day 60:

When we talk to others, one of the first questions we get is, "How is it living in the Ronald McDonald House?"

For most, taking an entire family and moving them into a one room house seems a bit insane. It can be. Instead of, "Clean up your room," it's become, "Clean up your area, space ... um, over here."

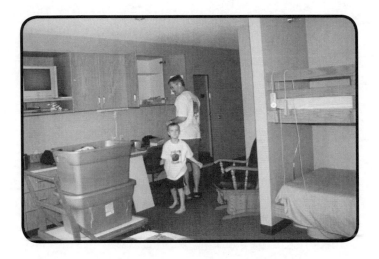

Our room contains a giant screen television (that's it on the shelf in the photo), two bunk–beds, a queen bed, a roll–a–way, and a bathroom; and we are also able to use the shared areas: a game room, a living room, a kitchen, a dining room, a kitchenette, and reading areas. The one thing you must concede in all of this is solitude.

This morning I was watching the news in the living room when one little boy was ready to go somewhere. As he stood in the doorway to his room screaming, "I'm ready! Let's go! I'm ready, I'm ready, I'm ready, I'm ready, " I was ready to take him wherever he wanted to go if he would concede the loudness to the morning news. It's at moments like these that you have to sit back, breathe, and remember that everyone in this house is here for a reason, and we're not all going to share the same style of living. Then I just have to remember how thankful we are to be in a place with the best care for Hannah. Then I hear the boy yelling some more, and I'm ready to really help him on his way. That's life in the Ronald McDonald House, though. Our room may be small at times, but we are doing just fine.

Top ten things that make life terrific when living in one room with your entire family:

10. You don't have to wonder if the shower is available.

9. You never fight for control of the television. You never had control to begin with.

8. When you have to go to the bathroom in the middle of the night and fall over something, severely damaging parts of your body you never

really knew existed, there's always someone there to ask if you're okay.

7. Everyone gets to take part in your conversation, so it's "family meeting time" all the time.

6. When you can't go to sleep, you can always ask, "Is anyone else awake?" Chances are, at ten p.m. at night, someone else is having trouble sleeping.

5. There are beds everywhere, just pick one!

4. It doesn't take long to clean.

3. You're hailed as king/queen when you leave the bathroom because now it's freed up for others.

2. Family movie night is every night!

And the number one thing that makes life terrific when living in one room with your entire family:

1. Bonding!

Hannah report: Counts are above super human. Thanks for the prayers. She has four more radiation treatments.

Turn and Burn

Day 62:
Once through the revolving door and into radiation

Hannah's arm is beginning to show signs of a farmers tan (just on the lower part of her arm), but it's a nasty sunburn instead. Those lasers can really do the trick. We met with our new radiologist, Dr. Nadia Laack (Lock), who spent some time with us today explaining the redness, swelling, and what is possibly happening inside her arm.

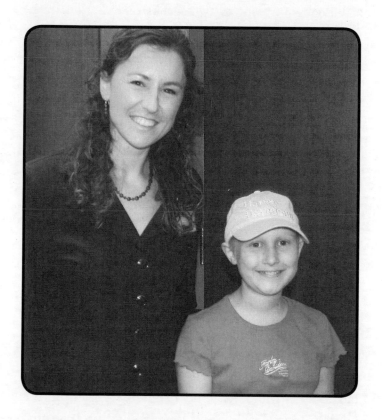

I had a new word to look up today: *fibrosis*. She was telling us that this is one thing that we need to keep an eye on as Hannah progresses through her treatments. She also explained that she would be a part of the surgery team in planning any possible radiation. If the surgeon is having trouble getting a negative field (which means the tumor has been completely removed), Dr. Laack could go in and zap it, giving it a dosage equivalent to two weeks of radiation treatments. As she explained in detail what is to come, we felt comforted being able to hear the path we must walk. She was reassuring the entire time. Hannah will have radiation follow up for quite some time to come because as Dr. Laack explains it, "We will be able to pick up signs that most wouldn't recognize." Here I thought we would be done once the entire treatment was complete.

My favorite part of our conversation came when Kim spoke up with, "What does the tumor look like inside?" After a brief chuckle, Dr. Laack responded with, "We can get you pictures during surgery." My adrenaline went up. How cool would that be? To be able to see what lies beneath and what will be no more. As it is, when Hannah's chemo treatments are complete, she will have her port removed and be able to take it home. In our family cancer group, one mother talked about how her child hangs the port from the Christmas tree each year. Don't know if we'll go that far, but I'm sure it will be available for conversations— much like a good flower assortment draws conversation as company sits around the table.

Hannah has two more radiation treatments to go! Pray that this is working.

In the Interest of Comedy

Day 63:
It's been a long two months of training. Did I say months? I stand corrected, weeks that felt like months. It seems like just yesterday when I wilted under pressure to the families' demand for entertainment and signed myself up for a tennis tournament.

Since that time, I've been engrossed in a "severe" training regimen that has me up by ten o'clock or so (depending on if the sunlight is peeking through the shade or not), on the courts by six–ish for a "two–hour workout" that lasts about forty–five minutes on a realistic scale, and back for a cool down in the room with a showing of *Hannah Montana*.

So far in the realm of training, I've discovered a very important thing: it's a good thing I'm doing this now (in Minnesota). There are no friends, no extended family, no one who knows me, and plenty of doctors and medical supplies to get me through. Although Max did mention tonight at dinner that, "Dad gets smoked tomorrow morning. It's gonna be cool!" With him on my side, how can I lose?

Training food is crucial: Royal Crown Cola with a Nutty Bar chaser. You know my opponent isn't even considering this type of training food—and that's where he went wrong.

My game plan is to get up early, go out strong, fake an injury, and leave the court limping. Years later around the fire ring…"I had that guy on the ropes. If it weren't for my big toe going into a hyperflex–tension–twist, the trophy would have been mine!"

Back up to game plan: win.

Double back up to game plan: just tell Max that I won so he'll stop referring to me as getting smoked.

Hannah update: She has been getting e–mails and loves to write back. Each morning she comes to me as I'm checking the e–mails myself and gives me the, "When are you going to be done?" Her radiation went well today, and she has one more to go.

The Games to Be

Day 64:

Brief tennis update: When I showed up at the tennis courts in the morning, two guys had already started a match. The rest of the courts lay empty. Strange, I thought, for a nine a.m. start time and to have no one around. But I am in Minnesota, and maybe things are done differently.

I walked into the clubhouse to announce my presence with authority when a high school kid tells me that there's no tennis on Saturday at the club. *No tennis on Saturday? Today's the tournament.* So I move onto the more logical question, "What about the tournament today?"

"Oh, that was last weekend. The dates were wrong on the flyer, but we did our best to get the word out."

Last weekend I was in prime form. I would have destroyed any opponent. Last weekend I had the abilities of Steve Austin, the Six Million Dollar Man.

The entire family was deflated like the ten–year-old tires on my bike after a long winter. We just sort of looked at one another in disbelief. Then the kids realized it was Saturday, and they were missing crucial cartoons. Crisis avoided, disappointment diverted, on with Saturday!

Out for the Week

Day 66:
I will be gone for the better part of this week. Our friends' baby boy, Evan, has passed away, and I'm heading home to be with the parents, Christine and James. Please pray for the family as they are most definitely struggling with the loss of their little boy. It's times like these that just leave me mystified as to why, yet at the same time, we ask God for his comfort and strength.

Friend Time

Day 70:
Back in Minnesota and ready to start round four of chemo.

I used to feel that home is home. Home is a town, a state, the home that you own. I have a new definition: home is where your family is located. The Ronald McDonald House has now become home. After being away this week, I can say that it's good to be back to my-one room, *Hannah Montana 24/7* home (although last night was a marathon of *Full House*). I'm waiting for a marathon of *Gilligan's Island!*

Hannah had a wonderful time with friends who drove out to visit this past week. It was a hair–styling, toe–painting, nature–seeing, city–dining, swim–swimming type of time. I know, what's *swim– swimming?* I needed an *–ing*—live with it. With her last radiation treatment on Monday and no shots or doctors Tuesday through Thursday, it was a great time.

Tonight we head back to Saint Mary's (bubble gum in hand and inspiration from a young girl named Sarah) to begin our last round before surgery. It's like the one last shot to do damage before they look at the tumor in the MRI. On the 26th we go through a series of scans and tests to determine the next stage (surgery) and how much of the tumor has been killed. It's one of those times that is both nerve–wracking and filled with the anticipation of moving forward at the same time.

I also have the Ronald McDonald House Ride this Sunday. With over a thousand riders participating, I'm just hoping to make new friends, not tip over, and represent all those biker–teachers out there. We're one of the tougher biker breeds 'cause we deal with kids all day.

Prayers: for Hannah, that she gets through her fourth round successfully and that her scans on the 26th come out as expected.

Danielle and the Puppy

Day 71:
There are some things to cover—so get comfortable or at least grab a second cup of coffee.

We entered the fourth round of chemotherapy last night and the first blow was ... no Amber. I had a bit of déjà vu all over again from the tennis tournament debacle.

Second wallop was no third floor. We would be staying on the second. You see, at St. Mary's, the third floor is for all the kids under eleven years of age. The second floor is for the older kids on up to adults. It's the equivalent of going from an elementary building right to the high school. We were hoping for the warm and fuzzy and ended up with, "Here's your room, we're booked solid upstairs," from the lady who appeared to be running the desk on her own this evening.

We did get another terrific nurse named Julia (no, not the *Julia* from "*Pretty Woman*"). She came in, and we immediately felt really comfortable with our new surroundings. She put us at ease by sharing one key item that we had overlooked. When you're on the teen floor, you don't hear babies crying all night long. You also have the teen game room, equipped with a giant screen television, foosball table, and lots of teen extras, such as computers, older board games (no more Chutes and Ladders), and more teen Playstation games. *Okay, this can't be that bad. It just means no more Candyland.* Julia also got right to work looking over Hannah's chart and talking to us about previous experiences we've had with treatments.

The third and fourth snafus came with Max coming down with an ear infection, and my development of something like a twelve–hour stomach flu. We ended up heading back to the House, giving Kim and Hannah some mother–daughter time. Even though Hannah's counts are okay now, she can't risk nurturing one of our viruses when she's at her lowest next week.

Enough with the pitfalls, the good news is that Hannah had a visitor today. Danielle, who has gone the cancer route herself (and just found out that her first after–treatment scans are clear), brought Hannah some wonderful "keep busy" items, as well as fashion accessories. The girls were able to enjoy a few short games and computer time together. As parents who have children with cancer, this is the picture you love to put in the memory bank and look at over and over because the smiles say it all.

Another fantastic part to the brighter side of things was hearing from the Hosbeins (Gary and Barb). Gary and Barb live right on the main beach in Saint Joseph overlooking Lake Michigan, so the kids have grown up knowing them as Beach Barb and Beach Gary. It's more of the unofficial replacement to any surname we might have for them.

Barb is always looking for neat little things to brighten up any day. Today she brought Hannah her very own puppy! Not a real one of course, but it did sit in its very own blanket–lined basket, and its stomach did move up and down with a breathing sound. If you're ever looking for the perfect pet to brighten up a hospital room, call Barb! Several nurses and doctors have taken a second, third, and fourth look before realizing that our sleeping dog is the perfect pet. Then they go and grab their coworkers to show them.

Hannah started her second batch this evening. She is doing really well through your prayers. We are very thankful for all your support.

1200 and Some

Day 72:

The big ride was today for the Ronald McDonald House. Last year they raised close to $80k and had just over one thousand bikes participate. The ride is one of the main benefits to raise money for the House. This year they have around 1,200 bikes, and I heard one of the event coordinators say that they just keep shattering records (referring to the amount of money raised).

Rain gear—check. Thunderstorms were rolling through the region, so I felt I should at least *carry* my gear. Although when riding, tough guy to tough guy, you would have to be facing hurricane–type rain before pulling off to the side to put on your rain gear when riding among a group of bikers. Rain is like road dirt...you expect to get some on you now and then (and it doesn't require a pull–over).

The ride was a bit intimidating at first. You are on your own for the actual ride—it was the parade to the Ronald McDonald House that we would do as a large group at the end of the day.

After signing up and receiving my packet, I made my way back out to the parking lot where many bikers had already gathered and were taking off at random. Inside my packet lay a single sheet, single spaced, Arial font type, size 12 (standard), paragraphed style directions. It's my belief that if AAA or Map Quest were to have started out with directions in this manner, each of their prospective board of directors would have been asked to retire early or to seek employment elsewhere. *How was I supposed to read the directions while traveling down the road in unknown territory?*

It was the sound of really loud pipes that snapped me out of my dilemma. *That's it! Follow the pack and don't get lost.* Once again, my high school diploma was paying off. I jumped on my bike, threw the wadded up directions deep into my right coat pocket, and slid in behind the loud guy. Things were looking up as we departed. I even had a couple of stragglers following me.

Half a mile down the road, I got caught at a red light, as Mr. "Hear My Chopper Roar" gunned it through the intersection. *Now I'm the lead bike; I can't be the lead bike. I wadded up the directions and stuffed them into my pocket. Not a good start. Maybe I should pull off to the side of the road and put on my rain gear?*

The remainder of the ride went well. We were in and out of mountains, cruising by rivers, and lost in the land of never–ending cornfields. In the mix of 1,200, you see all types of bikes and all types of people. It was a great day to be a people watcher and a bike admirer. I wish I could have shared it with all of my biking friends. It is definitely worth the drive to Minnesota to do again next year.

I picked up a passenger back at the Ronald McDonald House for the parade. Max got his first taste of the magnitude of being among all those bikers at full roar. I believe the words I heard over the rumble were, "Awesome! This is so awesome!" Kim and Hannah received a pass to leave the hospital (she was on liquids in between chemo) to walk the three blocks to see the bikes roll in from the parade route. Hannah was drained by the experience but excited to see all the bikes—probably almost as excited as Max and I were to spot them in the crowd.

I know the ride for Hannah is coming up back in Michigan next weekend. I wish everyone safe travels—shiny side up. I'll be thinking of you.

Move It or Lose It

Day 73:
From biker to mover, we have officially received a long–term room. The Ronald McDonald House only has six out of forty–two rooms that are deemed long–term. What's long–term you ask? Here's the upgrade: *two rooms, two televisions, a small refrigerator, microwave, two sinks, and a couch.*

Hannah was really ready to get out of the hospital today after her fourth round concluded. As we sat and watched the clock tick past noon, her nurse, Sara, informed us that Zofran was on the way, and then we would be released—wahoo! Zofran is the medicine that keeps her stomach calm as her body adjusts to the attack from the chemo. Feeling fairly confident, Hannah requested a trip to Buffalo Wild Wings (darn the luck).

Moving was a bit more challenging than last time since losing our "one guy and a cart" to his friends back in Michigan. The last move, Kim took care of packing, Sam handled moving, and I rounded out the combo with the unpacking. With no middle Sam–man in the mix, we were left completely disorganized. Hannah tried to jump in and was successful for about an hour, but she became tired quickly, so a day off was necessary.

This week we have shots beginning tomorrow. Grandpa Kelly needs to pry open that wallet again. By Thursday evening we should know what the treatments have done to the tumor and the game plan for surgery.

Peace and prayers.

In the Dark

Day 74:
With the move finalized, the finishing touches were done as Kim put up the photo wall today. Of course, there are still photos out there that we haven't received

yet, not that I'm throwing out electronic guilt or anything.

Staying in our new room brought about new experiences last night. Kim likes to call the place "The Cave," mainly because it's in the back of the building with our two windows looking out on a wall covered in ivy. This, of course, is in contrast to our street–view bay window, which always had action going on and streetlights at night. *The Cave* was truly dark when we shut off the lights. Normally this would be a good thing, but when you're used to everyone being up throughout the night to use the bathroom, it creates banging issues.

Our wonderful late–night walks stem from Hannah staying hydrated. I thought I drank quite a bit of water in my daily routine, but for some reason her hydration is tied directly into everyone's bladder growth, kind of like yawning—one person does it and the rest join in.

So we lay there … in the pitch black. "What are we going to do?" Kim questions, probably making the first move in order to be the one to stay in bed, while I get up to figure something out.

"I don't know," was my reply, followed by a brief silence, thinking I would hear a deep sigh out of her as she got up to find some light to turn on.

Silence, followed by a whole lot of nothingness.

"Well?" was her response. That's the ultimate card any wife can play in the game of "Who Gets out of

Bed First?" When you get the "*well,*" you might as well come to grips with the terms of the game: you're the guy, and it's your job to take care of anything electrical in the House (even if it means finding the switch and risking toe injury).

Up I went. I did the foot shuffle to insure limited foot pain upon contact and found the switch. Of course, it was the wrong switch. The whole process was about a ten–minute ordeal that ended with the words: "Just get in bed and forget it. We'll be fine."

Forget it. I've devoted my *now* existence to this problem. How would I sleep? *Forget it* was not part of the solution. I flipped switches, tested angles of lighting, and did everything short of a total rewire on our two–room mansion.

Nothing worked.

Tomorrow would be my day of *Return to Glory* (a little something for those Irish fans out there), I assured myself. Back to bed I went, happy to lay my head on my pillow.

"I'm hot. Is the air on?" Kim mentions casually.

Hannah woke this morning with her exploits of spelunking to the bathroom last night. "Dad, what are you going to do about it?" Hannah emphasized the need for more light at night in order to navigate the new territory.

Who sang the song "In the Dark"? (No fair using iTunes either). First person to respond gets my respect and a little something in their stocking at Christmas.

An All Day Event–Here We Go

Day 75:
First things first—night light is installed!

Okay, now that I have that monkey off my back, we just want to share with everyone that we appreciate your prayers and support. Tomorrow is one of those moments that you know to be a "fork in the road." As we go through the scans in the morning and await the results late afternoon, we can't bluff our way through it and say that we feel absolutely at peace. Our stomachs are in knots, our hopes are on edge, and our prayers are being said hourly. We place our trust in God and his plan for Hannah, yet we may not be thrilled with the choice of path.

As you have followed our journey from day one to day seventy–five, this is the time we have waited for: the point at which we find out if the chemo and radiation have done their part to insure that the cancer has not spread and for the surgeons to move to the next phase. Through your prayers we will move forward and be strong.

Peace and prayers.

Bugs Administers CT

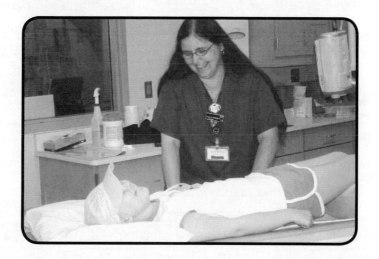

Day 76:

I haven't seen six a.m. for quite a while, but we were up early to get to the Mayo Clinic for an MRI, a CT scan, and blood work. The good thing about getting up early is ... nothing.

In the afternoon, we had visits with the hand specialist (reconstruction doctor), the tumor specialist (surgeon), and the radiologist (the radiologist).

First the good news: No spreading of the cancer cells to the lungs. We were told that they didn't do a bone scan this time because they wanted to see the lungs first. If the cancer were to spread, it would go there first.

The tumor itself had not decreased in size, and they won't know if the radiation and chemo have done the trick until they get in there and take it out. The plan is to have the surgeon go in and cut out all tumor–looking material and check for margins as he goes. Simply put, he checks for good and bad tissue.

The radiologist will perform further radiation on the parts that have been in contact with the tumor to ensure a clean field. Right now, the median (middle) nerve might possibly be spared. If it is, she will put in tubes for further radiation.

The reconstruction specialist is planning for the loss of two out of the three major nerves in the forearm. He plans on using nerves from Hannah's legs to rebuild one nerve, and he has thoughts of using Axogen Nerve Regeneration (http://www.axogeninc.com/). It's a new treatment that he says should work in theory. He hasn't used it on a patient yet, so Hannah will become the first (if it's needed). He also mentioned taking muscles from other parts of her body, along with skin, for grafting. I was still stuck on comprehending the Axogen Theory and missed most of the grafting phase. All I know is it's going to be a procedure.

The surgery is scheduled for August 14. We will have one more round of meetings with the doctors to confirm the plan and to ask last minute questions the day before.

Highlights of the day: *Bugs* (pictured above) was an 1860s baseball player that we watched with the Simpson family over the Rochesterfest days. She plays in the league as a regular and loves hassling the opponents and the umpire. She carries many quarters with her because every time she does or says something inappropriate, she gets fined two bits. With her sense of humor, she gets fined a lot. Our CT scan was the most enjoyable. What should have been about five minutes lasted fifteen because we couldn't stop talking with her.

Thank you so much for the thoughts, prayers, and support.

Keep reading.

And the Beat Goes On

Day 77:

Today we met with our oncologist to go over Hannah's recent blood work and her overall health after chemo. We began discussing the surgery and all that it involved (removal of the tumor, possible radiation, and reconstruction options). That's when the wheels came off the bus.

Our oncologist is considered the "primary" when it comes to Hannah's overall treatment. She feels that the reconstruction is best done after all chemo and radiation have taken their course (which would put us somewhere in November). She also wanted to stay on the national protocol. If you deviate from the protocol then you can no longer submit your findings and be a part of the national protocol.

Trying to sort out how things are to go was quite a task, mainly because I think the doctors were trying to sort it out themselves. As parents we need things black and white, laid out in front of us like a flow chart. The only problem was our flow chart was not linear because of the multiple issues faced by the different department doctors working with Hannah.

Well, that's not what the others were planning. We were supposed to have removal and reconstruction at the same time.

No, that's not right. We are supposed to have removal, then radiation, then reconstruction.

Nope. That's not right either. Reconstruction might have to be a week later.

Wrong again! Darn it! It's removal, radiation, chemotherapy, then reconstruction months later. *That could be the final plan, but hang on, the doctors will have to talk it through.*

We left the office feeling like leaves in a windstorm. We're just waiting to see which way we'll be blown. We were told that they would all get together and hash out the best plan for Hannah, according to her protocol. We've gotten to know each specialty doctor and feel confident that they will make the best decision for Hannah. This is a time for us to step back, be patient, and listen.

Ride for Hannah is tomorrow. "I wish I could be there," Hannah told me, after finding out that the Storm Team (her travel basketball team), family, friends, and bikers were going to be there. "We all would love to be there," I assured her. Enjoy the ride, the fellowship, and be safe. Most importantly, let me know if Eight Ball (my good friend and riding partner, Tim Reynolds) polished his chrome for the ride.

Peace and prayers and shiny side up (for all those bikers who are reading).

Another Day in the Sota

Day 79:

If you were to look up "great day" in the medical journals, it would say *Harley Davidson*, but right below that would be the words *Kelly Family, July 29th*. It was one of those days that just ran from one good thing to another.

It all began with a phone call days ago. "Would you like visitors?" was the question.

Hannah has been corresponding with a number of people, but Sami and her mom, Cheri, had been following Hannah and our stories and just developed a connectedness. Sami (aka: Samantha) had gone through her own bout with medical procedures, so she has some personal insight into what Hannah is going through. Sami and Hannah had been writing for a little bit but had never met—even though we probably live ten miles apart back home. I had Sami's older brother, Jacob, as a fifth grader. I still remember Sami coming up to me in the hallway at school and asking me if I could tell her brother to be nicer to her. I had no problems doing that. Jacob was a great kid, but like most brothers had a love of torturing sibling sisters. I also had Sami in youth basketball, but even with the connection I had, Hannah had no idea who she was. They never had the chance to meet—until now.

We spent time talking, laughing, and touring the House and Rochester. It was one of those visits when you meet someone for the first time, but it feels like you are sitting down with old friends. "I wish they could have stayed longer. They were really nice, and Sami's mom was crazy," Hannah remarked as they left. By the way, crazy is good coming from a ten–year–old.

After our friends left, I had the opportunity to run out to a local high school and watch my new friend, Steve, work a basketball clinic. One of my favorite things to do as a coach is to pick up new ideas and talk basketball with other coaches. I was getting my basketball fix for the day, and it felt wonderful.

Upon returning to the RMH (Ronald McDonald House), I learned that Kim and her newfound friend, Claudia (from Guatemala), had been out walking the hills of Rochester. The two love to spend time talking with one another and sharing their respective lifestyles and countries. Claudia is an energetic lady who is starting a women's magazine and would like Kim to write for her. Once Kim stopped laughing, she deferred the writing to me. The only problem is that Claudia needs women writing the articles.

Let's recap: We had visitors from Michigan, I got in some b–ball, and Kim's developing a new career in international journalism.

Same Day, Different Topic

Day 80:
I should get a double bonus for writing twice in one day. Technically, last night's writing was at 12:13 a.m. on July 30. What would a double bonus entail? I have no idea since I wouldn't even know what a bonus would look like for writing down life in the Sota.

Kim often asks, after the lid to the Mac Book shuts, "What could you possibly write about?"

Truthfully, sometimes I sit down and just stare at the screen as my eyes slowly gloss over, head slamming to the counter with a thud, and that's when it hits me (no, not the counter, the idea of what to write about). Other days, we have so many things going on, I feel as if I could write forever (but I try not to in order to keep it short and simple). No matter what, though, we try to include what's happening in the world of Mayo, Minnesota, and Hannah.

Tomorrow we're up early for blood work, followed by a visit with our oncologist. We're hoping some decisions have been made in regard to Hannah's next step.

Our time over the next week will be filled with activities just to keep the downtime at a minimum. Fortunately, they have the county fair this week; unfortunately, this is not the week to have Hannah out and about.

She doesn't talk much about her surgery other than saying, "Can we not talk about it? It makes me nervous." We keep reassuring her that she'll be sound asleep through the whole thing, but I think it's more of the thoughts of what's to come after surgery. Kim and I can't help but think about the after.

Our number one prayer is that they get negative margins, but our radiologist and oncologist feel that the sarcoma and the fibromatosis (the original benign tumor) have contacted so much, that negative margins might be unlikely. A margin is the distance between the tumor and the edge of the tissue. When you reach negative margins you have no more cancer tissue in connection with the healthy tissue. I haven't heard of any other cancer patient who had their radiologist in on the surgery. Of course, now that I think about it, we didn't see other cancer kids receiving radiation either.

Our other big question is the trade off of post-poning reconstruction. We're not sure if that means her right arm and hand will become immobile for the duration of treatment or to what it will lead. Hopefully our meeting tomorrow will answer some questions that always seem to pop up when we're *not* in front of the doctors.

Keep praying, keep reading.

Peace and prayers.

Limb Salvage

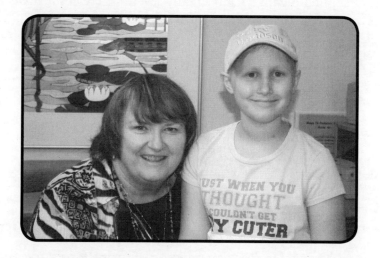

This is Donna. She shared her terrier and snoodle dogs with us today. They looked awfully cute, but she said when they eat her remote controls, the carpet, and her glasses, they don't seem so cute. Donna was one of Hannah's go–to–gals in the pediatric oncology department.

Day 81:
I found out one crucial piece of "life" information this morning as we got up to ready ourselves for a busy morning at the Mayo Clinic: our body clocks are going to need several weeks to adjust back to E.S.T. We had to get up at six–thirty this morning, and it was as pleasant as pulling cactus from the desert without gloves. The entire time I spent prying open an eyelid, I kept telling myself, "It's really seven–thirty. It's really seven–thirty." Of course, going to bed at twelve–thirty wasn't a wise decision.

We made it to the Mayo right on schedule—five minutes late for our appointment (which is right on time for us). Hannah had to have her port accessed for the blood draw. She usually keeps accessed in case the blood work comes back and shows that she needs a transfusion (which has happened only once). After a brief blood draw, we headed to Caribou for coffee and donuts (probably not the healthiest diet when at the Mayo).

Seeing Dr. Rodriguez was a surprise for us. We had originally been scheduled to see Donna, the nurse practitioner; however, we received a call yesterday saying that the doctor wants to see us. I chalked it up to hammering out the surgical procedures that we were to follow. I was wrong (kind of).

Dr. Rodriguez started the conversation with, "I have some concerns." *Oh no, this can't be good.*

The doctors did have a conversation about Hannah, but it didn't necessarily revolve around the order of procedures. Instead they discussed margins (aka: getting all the cancer out). She is not comfortable with the fact that the tumor has not shrunken at all and is equally concerned about whether the radiation and chemo have affected it. This was one of those *rare* conversations we had back in April/May. *It would be rare for the tumor to not respond.*

Dr. Rodriguez wants to take all precautions, which take into consideration Hannah's life over "limb salvage" (that's what they call it rather than "saving her arm"). So amputation is back on the table. It was never really gone, just pushed off to a far corner.

The surgeon, Dr. Shives, mentioned that the pathologist will be able to tell exactly how much of the tumor was destroyed once they remove it. He mentioned it may be 90 percent, or it could be 30 percent. When I mentioned percentages to Dr. R. and asked what would be acceptable for her, she said that the percentage of dead tumor would have to be very close to 100 percent in order to move forward with limb salvage. Her concern is that if the tumor is not dead, then the radiation and the chemo weren't 100 percent effective; therefore, microscopic cancer cells could survive and bring about recurrence or metastasize (move) to the lungs. The oncology team, along with the national group, will be discussing acceptable percentages over the next week. Personally, I'm more in line with the 100 percent number rather than playing the odds.

Hannah began the conversation really, really nervously, but eventually became her normal, smiling self. She realizes the danger if the tumor has not been fully destroyed. She doesn't really care for the amputation option, but we've been talking about it from the beginning.

We wrapped up the morning with her GCSF (granulocyte colony–stimulating factor) shot with Deena.

We're off to the county fair this afternoon for fair food!

Pray for the 100 percent, and if that's not his will, then that amputation and transition go smoothly.

Peace and prayers.

August

Flying High

Day 83:

I spent most of my day tied up in download limbo. Ever try and take the shortcut by just clicking on the download button? *How hard could it be, right? I'm connected to high speed. I don't have to wait for a shipment. I don't even have to pay for shipping. It's all good in the world of technology.*

I was up until two in the morning after two unsuccessful downloads (each taking about an hour). All I wanted was to update my camera software. Okay, I got a late start on it, but two a.m.—seriously. It has to be easier. Good thing I like technology and find it to be helpful most times, otherwise I would have plans for my laptop as a Frisbee.

I got up this morning, and by five p.m. this evening I had that laptop humming like a kid with cheeks stuffed with the finest confection from a chocolate factory. Five downloads, one technical call, three service calls, one sales call, a great deal of elevator music, and a simple plug in. I now have a photo program. I can hear your excitement building as you think, *Dave's gone pro photographer with his filters and color enhancements.* You may be right. More importantly, I now get to log more computer time in the family realm because I hold photo enhancement priority. I know, a lot of work for a little edge.

These past few days have been busy. The county fair is taking place this week. If you know our family, its sole purpose in August revolves around fair food.

While the Olmstead County Fair has its pleasant points, I give the Berrien County Fair (in Michigan) the nod. Although, I don't recall the bungee jumping that Max found and couldn't pass by. It was awesome to see him shoot about two stories high and overlook the fairgrounds.

After hearing that all of the bikers in the Ride for Hannah received a God Strong wristband, we picked up bands of our own. The bands from the ride are based on Ephesians 6:10–11. What a terrific message for others to carry. We have ours being sent out thanks to Vicar Rod. Kim and I were so moved by the sentiment and the message that we headed to the nearest Christian store.

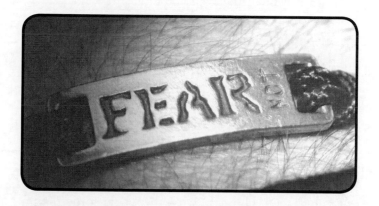

I wanted a band that would signify this experience for our family. I think I found the perfect one. It says simply Fear Not.

> I took you from the ends of the earth, from its farthest corners I called you. I said, "You are my servant"; I have chosen you and not rejected you. So do not fear, for I am with you; do not be dismayed, for I am your God. I will strengthen you and help you; I will uphold you with my righteous right hand.
>
> Isaiah 41:9–10 (NIV)

The other message I get from the wristband is:

> And David said to Solomon his son, "Be strong
> and of good courage, and do it: Fear not, nor be
> dismayed: for the LORD God, even my God, will
> be with thee; he will not fail thee, nor forsake
> thee, until thou hast finished all the work for the
> service of the LORD."
>
> 1 Chronicles 28:20 (NIV)

Between Fear Not and God Strong, I will be reminded daily of God's love and His promise. The messages are clear and powerful. Kim and Sam both got one as well. Hannah, well, she wants something a bit more girly looking. So we'll keep looking.

Tomorrow we are participating in a Relay for Life with the Hucke family in Kasson, Minnesota. They and their group (including us) get to walk the first lap. I asked Danielle (their daughter who recently finished with her cancer treatment) what would I get if I came in first. "What?" was her reply. She needs to get to know me better. I hope to capture some pictures and put my marathon download software to work.

Peace and prayers. Surgery in twelve days.

Face It

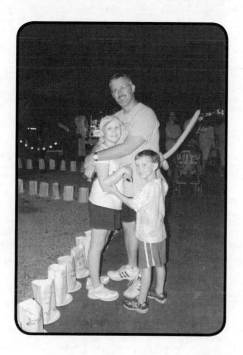

Day 84:

It was a tough day in terms of facing cancer. There are many different levels at which we've had to face cancer: the diagnosis, telling family and friends, the hospital visits, the writing, the daily issues that come with cancer, and now... Relay for Life.

I have done many fundraisers in the past (mainly through motorcycle rides), and it always felt good to know that we were raising money for an important cause. I even participated in a Relay for Life years back. I showed up and put in my two hours or so of track walking. The word *caretaker* came up several times tonight, and I suppose that's the role that I felt comfortable playing. I was the caretaker, the one who raised money for those who needed it. It wasn't supposed to be for my family or me. Tonight put that in a different perspective for me.

When I first saw Hannah's luminary on the side of the track, I had a flood of emotions that were bouncing all over the gamut: anger, sadness, hopefulness, tranquility, weakness, and most of all, a bit of helplessness.

I couldn't bring myself to ask Hannah how she felt. After all, here we were, surrounded by people who had beaten cancer and others who had lost a loved one. We were right there in the middle, and I had no clue how an eleven–year–old would respond or think of it all.

The first lap is for survivors. Dawn asked Kim and our family to join everyone in the walk. I took one look at Kim, with tears streaming down her face, and it was just about all I could do to not go there myself. I knew exactly what she was going through. It was at that moment that Dawn told her that Hannah is a survivor. She's just in the middle of the battle, but she's surviving. That's all it took, and they were out in the group ready for the walk.

Steve, Dawn, Danielle, and Collin (our adoptive family and friends) shared their story of Danielle with the entire relay crowd. The strength they drew from all of those who supported them was very powerful to witness. It took one line in their story to change one part of how I had been feeling about facing cancer: the idea of letting others care for you. *I don't want to be taken care of, I want to be the one to help others.* But that's not where I am at now. We, as a family, are not yet where we can begin to take care of others. We have to let others care for us. We have each other; we have you; and we have faith. We can face cancer. We can face it together.

Although I didn't really care for the Relay for Life because it put cancer in front of me again, it was good to go through because it made me *face cancer.* Does that make sense?

Each time I face it, I become stronger ... we become stronger. We become less fearful. We become more determined. I look forward to taking the first lap with Hannah next year. Just as the Huckes enjoyed their lap with Danielle and others, we will do it with all of our friends and family.

Peace and prayers. We ask for 100 percent of the tumor to be dead and for a negative field during surgery on the fourteenth of this month.

Punchy or Just Slow

Day 85:

Who ordered the *Rocky* marathon on cable? I know it had to have been through prayer because the one thing everybody needs on a rainy day is *Rocky I, II, III, IV, and V!*

One of my favorite lines of all times comes in *Rocky II* when Apollo taunts Rocky over and over to get him to fight a second time. It gets to the point where Mickey can't take it anymore and heads over to Rocky's house to let him know that they should accept the fight. Okay, so now that you recall the scene, here's the line:

"I tink we should knock his block off," Mickey states in his gruff voice.

"Absoluly," is Rocky's reply in his biggest slurred, post–Vicodin state.

The second favorite line comes in *Rocky II* as well, right in the beginning when Rocky's at the hospital and journalists are all around him:

"Rocky! What were your thoughts when going into that last round?"

"I wished I woulda finished school."

It's the little things in life. Thanks for the prayers.

Hola

Day 87:

The one thing about living at the RMH is that you never are far from someone's story.

Rodrigo and his mom, Claudia, are from Guatemala. Rodrigo was given the option of amputation by the oncologists in his homeland. This wasn't acceptable to his family, who began a worldwide search for another answer. It was Mayo Clinic, and Dr. Shives, who answered her e–mail with the opportunity to save the leg.

Rodrigo and Claudia began back in the winter of '06 with straight surgery to remove the cancer. His entire femur was removed and reconstruction begun. This trip was a month–long rehab and more reconstruction.

"It's amazing the things the doctors can do," she recalls.

We just returned from our second trip to the Mall of America. Rodrigo was tired from walking on crutches, but the fact was, he was still doing it with two legs.

We see amazing things on a daily basis here at the House. Some people we get to know intimately; we hear the stories of others through common room chats. Yet it's all the same thread that runs through each story: that of children who have struggles that they must overcome and the prayers they say each and every night before their heads hit the pillow. It's a story of healing and hope.

We have made good friends in Rodrigo and his mom. They have become a part of our lives as we have become part of theirs. There's something about the House that makes you feel at ease sharing your life with others. It's the common bond of our children that brings us close in a short amount of time. With e–mails and addresses exchanged, we have made a friendship that will stretch beyond the national borders.

As Claudia would say, "It is good. Very good."

Girl Time

Day 88:
Tonight was our cancer support group (Brighter Tomorrows), which meets every first Tuesday of the month (if you're in the area). I believe I told you about the group already, but just in case you forgot, the group is made up of parents with children who have survived cancer, those who are going through it, and some who are at the beginning.

We had a guest speaker who talked about alternative medicine: acupuncture, massage, yoga, and meditation, etc. The idea is to provide patients and caregivers, also known as the parents, a chance to reduce the stress in their lives and to learn how to take care of themselves. When he mentioned massage I was hoping that he was going to follow it with free coupons or passes or something. No such luck.

It didn't take long for me to lean into Kim and start to say, *"I think we need this right now!"* Kim looked at me with a quick glance and replied, "I know."

We never really considered the added stress that comes with cancer care, but it explains a lot. For instance, I now have gray hair. I know... shocker.

During our group, Hannah enjoys the parent time because it means that she has her time with the other kids.

All of these young ladies (because it's a group of girls) have been through the cancer experience, which makes them the number one resource for Hannah—and they have a lot of fun, too. Shanna seems to be one of the main group leaders for the kids. "Mom and Dad, this is Shanna... she's a dancer," Hannah introduced Shanna to us.

"I didn't say I was a dancer," Shanna chuckled as she placed a hand on her amputated leg (where the cancer had grown when she was eight years old), "I said I had cancer!"

"What? I thought you said you were a dancer." Hannah and the others got a good laugh out of the confusion. Shanna quickly became the cancer dancer girl.

Other news from today: We heard from one of our doctors. It seems that the group has spent many hours discussing Hannah and the best way to proceed with her. They have a *planner* who helps them coordinate the various groups that will be working on Hannah come Tuesday.

From what I understand, the issue of the potentially dead tumor is important, but not as important as we once thought. If amputation does have to happen, the chance of the cancer spreading still exists. Which means that the real question becomes: "How salvageable is the arm?" As for radiation procedures, they will be done after surgery is complete. Hannah will be transported downtown to the clinic where they will give her the radiation and then back to the hospital. As for reconstruction, we will wait until Monday to meet with the other doctors to hear what the overall plan is. If they can meet the deadline for the next chemotherapy, then I believe we will have reconstruction done right after radiation.

Kim wasn't around when the phone call came in, but apparently my big question of, "Do we have to get up early on Tuesday for the surgery?", although semi–important to me, was not among the list of critical questions that I should have asked. I could really have used a massage at that particular point in time.

In the meantime, the girls have declared it party time and intend on getting in movies, swimming, and fun before next Monday.

Wheelchair and Child Life

Day 89:

Hannah was so excited today to receive her American Girl Doll order, which contained a wheel chair and crutches for her doll. I suppose you can see where her mindset is. I was personally thinking of ordering a growler from the Livery, possibly for our return trip to Michigan.

Hannah also had a chance to talk with Kim, the child life specialist at the RMH. Kim and Hannah were able to talk about all of those things that possibly run through the minds of kids before they undergo big procedures. It was another great connection for Hannah. As you can see, she came back to the room and prepared Danielle for a little procedure as well. Danielle looks pretty excited about the whole thing.

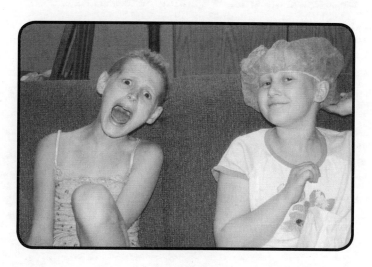

We have four more days to get in all the fun we can before surgery. It's almost the reverse countdown before Christmas. We know we'll be hospital bound for a few weeks. Tomorrow the guys head to the ball field while the girls make plans for a girl movie.

Thank you so much for your prayers, your concerns, and reading.

Peace and prayers–The Kelly's

It's a Minni World

Day 92:

Two days ago, when coming home from the local Honkers baseball game, we were given tickets to the Minnesota Vikings preseason opener against the St. Louis Rams. There were just two tickets. That night there was a question of whom to take.

Naturally I had secured my ticket because I was the guy with the car keys.

Hannah wasn't interested. Kim wanted to go but wasn't sure after going to an arena football game for our anniversary. I know, ladies, what was your husband thinking by taking you to a nice dinner, giving you flowers, and maybe even doing some dancing when you could have been at arena football? She thought she could pass on the experience.

So it was down to Sam and Max. One wanted to go to see the game; the other wanted to go because there might be cotton candy and ring pops. I left it open for the evening. After all, I had the whole next morning to figure out a fair way of whom to take.

The very next morning there was a knock at the door. Kim and I looked at one another. "Company at our palace?"

It turned out to be Patty, the manager, with four more tickets to the game. One, two, three, four, five, six! This was fantastic. We had enough for everyone plus a guest! Is that considered God's timing when you think about the night before?

The game itself was exciting, but it was even more so when you add the crowd participation, which roared around us as the Viking fans kicked their enthusiasm into overdrive. None of us has ever been to a professional game before, but I now know why people are sitting at a football game in freezing weather while I'm at home on my couch. It's a completely different experience to be there in person rooting on your team. Although I didn't really have a *team* on this go around, I now have a desire to get Bears tickets.

The game was a lot of fun and was tied at ten apiece going into the last minute and a half. Two seconds left, the Rams marched down the field, and thanks to the Vikings defensive coordinator calling for a loose zone to avoid the long ball, the Rams kicked a field goal, and won the game by three points. I don't think the Viking fans would have taken it so hard if it weren't for their kicker missing a thirty–plus–yard try right before the Rams' final push and score.

After the game we were confronted with more trying times equal to that of the field goal loss. We were in a city with no GPS, no map, a lot of one–way streets, multiple highway systems, and hostile Viking fans in cars. We had no plans for getting out.

We started by driving parallel to the highway with a general sense of which way was east, but there was no onramp in sight. It reminded me a great deal of our cancer experience. You start in a general direction and can see that you're moving forward, but you're not quite sure where it will take you.

Here we were, so close to the road that we needed to be on, yet had no way of getting on. I was so close that I could see the whites of the drivers' eyes. It was the Battle of Bunker Hill in modern times. Yet as I drove down the road, a wall slowly rose up out of the ground, growing ever higher, obscuring my view, and cutting the crew and me off from our destined direction.

We ended up cruising through neighborhoods that we had no business being in, hitting dead ends, and saying famous quotes like, "Hey, we've seen this before," "Look, there's the city over there," and "I'm hungry. Can we eat soon?"

I obviously made it back; otherwise, I wouldn't be writing this. What we did was make our way back to "start." "Someone, everyone, start looking for angry

Vikings and a big dome building." The one thing about being lost is that you always know from where you started. We made our way back to the Metrodome, and it took us about five minutes and one U–turn before we were cruising down the right highway, watching the wall rise up, separating us from our memories of "lock the doors."

Connected

Day 93:
Yesterday, the bike ride.

Today, making the connection.

Before even arriving in Minnesota, we had heard about a congregation called Trinity Lutheran Church. It was the home church of a vicar back in St. Joseph.

When we arrived in Minnesota, we began receiving heartfelt cards from the members of Trinity. Again it was God's hand reaching out to us through people whom we didn't know. Through Vicar Hatteburg, the people of Trinity came to know our family and began praying for us and sending cards/care packages.

Trinity is located in the countryside near the little town of Waltham. As described by the vicar in a letter, "If you blink, you'll miss it." He wasn't far off. We turned down a country road where a road sign read "thirty m.p.h."

"Strange, I don't see a town. Oh wait, there it is," I said, pointing at a two–road community with a park.

We had arrived in Waltham. Ten seconds later, we were moving past it.

The members of Trinity made walking through their door feel as if we had been there before. This small church felt inviting, warm, and most importantly for us, it felt like home. The other thing that really impressed me was the singing. Wow, could these people put a hymn together. If there was ever a place for congregations to go for singing lessons, this would be the place.

Pastor Kuddes delivered the message that we needed to hear.

> Then Jesus said to his disciples: Therefore I tell you, do not worry about your life, what you will eat; or about your body, what you will wear. Life is more than food, and the body more than clothes. Consider the ravens: They do not sow or reap, they have no storeroom or barn; yet God feeds them. And how much more valuable you are than birds! Who of you by worrying can add a single hour to his life? Since you cannot to this very little thing, why do you worry about the rest?
>
> Luke 12:22–26 (NIV)

It was one that warranted reading again once I got back to the RMH. Following the service, the congregation spent time with our family. I even met a number of bikers among the congregation and hope to get in a ride with the Trinity bikers. This visit couldn't have come at a better time.

We spent the rest of the afternoon with Pastor Kuddes and his family. It was a very relaxing and enjoyable time with a little cookout and plenty of visiting. We now have a deeper connection to our Minnesota church family and understand what Vicar Hatteburg means when he talks about the wonderful people of Trinity.

Tomorrow we meet with more doctors in the afternoon to hopefully gain a better understanding of what lies ahead on Tuesday. I should have news by tomorrow evening.

That's the Plan, Stan!

Day 94:
Tonight, anytime between eight–thirty and midnight, we make the call and receive our check–in time for surgery tomorrow. That was the easy part of the instructions on the down low (DL—see kids, I'm learning the hip terms) for today.

We met with the doctors, Bishop and Shin, who will be taking notes during the surgery and preparing for possible reconstruction. It seems that the overall plan will go something like this: surgery tomorrow to remove the tumor and a majority of muscle, tendons, nerves, and the old fibromatosis. After removing the tumor, Dr. Shives, our tumor specialist, will confer with Dr. Rodriguez, our pediatric oncologist. Between the two of them, they will decide whether to continue forward with reconstruction or to move into amputation. We will also have Dr. Laack, our radiologist, there to prepare for the insertion of the tubes. Should reconstruction be the next step, she will radiate the arm on Wednesday. Have I lost anyone yet?

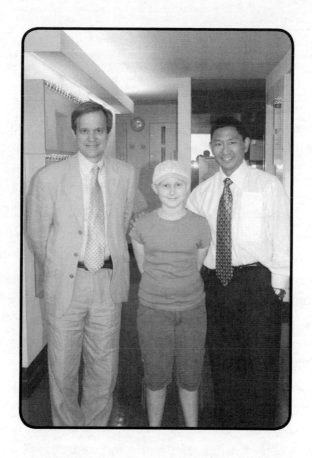

Dr. Bishop and Dr. Shin ran through multiple plans with us today. It was like one big flow chart being laid out..."If this happens, then we can do this. If this is cut out, then we can replace with either this or that."

They covered both nerve and muscle reconstruction, as well as went over various tendon options and future movement. What it came down to when all was said and done is that Hannah will have about a year or more of rehab in which her movement will gradually build back, or possibly not, depending on the amount of damage done by removing the tumor. There's always the uncertainty of what's to come—as we've become experts at realizing. What is good is that both Dr. Shin and Dr. Bishop will be in the operating room watching Dr. Shives tomorrow. Then, if the plan is to move forward with limb salvage and reconstruction, Hannah will receive radiation from Dr. Laack on Wednesday, and the two hand specialists will operate on Thursday. So Dr. Shin and Dr. Bishop will have a full day to discuss which plans they want to follow. It also gives Hannah a break, making the process a two-surgery deal rather than one long, long day. Not that she'll remember much with all the medicine that she'll be receiving.

So, for tonight, we swim, eat, and swim some more! Hannah's being a trooper. She wants to go eat wings just in case her arm's amputated. She's not sure how she'll eat wings with only one hand. I think we'll figure out a way.

We appreciate your prayers.

> You gave me life and showed me kindness, and in your province watched over my spirit.
>
> Job 10:12 (NIV)

Go Time

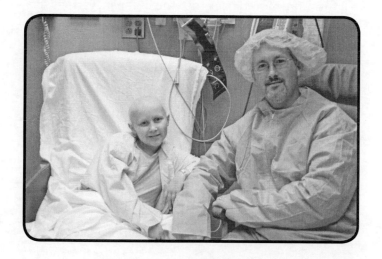

Do not be anxious about anything, but in everything, by prayer and petition, with thanksgiving,
present your requests to God. And the peace of
God, which transcends all understanding, will
guard your hearts and minds in Christ Jesus.

Philippians, 4:6–7 (NIV)

Day 95:

8:35: Five a.m. comes quickly when you go to sleep at
two, but in the scheme of things, that's small potatoes.
We had to arrive at the hospital by six–fifteen to begin
the admission process, which entails being admitted
to the hospital, going through check–in on the sur-

gery floor, and getting into the bull pen (aka: the prep area).

Once we moved back into the bull pen, various services began their stop–by visits to go over procedures and questions. By services, I'm referring to the surgeons, anesthesiologists, and operating–room nurses.

Hannah also had the usual vital signs and questions checked prior to going back: "Your name is … ? You're having what done today? Your doctors are … ?" Hannah has to answer these over and over again to avoid any mistakes. It makes sense after walking back to the operating room (O.R.) where everyone is dressed in blue and wearing masks.

Having the chance to go back to the operating room with Hannah was awesome! The operating rooms are packed with equipment and about fifteen to twenty various people in motion getting things ready. Hannah fell asleep within seconds of getting the gas, and my time in the O.R. was concluded, although I offered to stay.

We have been put in Hannah's hospital room while she's in surgery. Being back in her hospital room beats sitting in a waiting room any day. We can relax a little more, if that's really possible at a time like this. Our next step is to wait, pray, and wait some more.

8:50: Our nurse communicator just stopped by to give us the update. The surgery started at eight forty–five. She said that sometimes the doctor calls the room to talk to us; sometimes he asks to see us in person (they are on the floor below us). Sometimes Dr. Shives lets the parents view the tumor. Kim passed on that offer, but I'd like to see what was in there. She will contact us periodically to give us an update as the procedure progresses.

10:30: The communication nurse called the room. They have completed Hannah's surgery, and she will be moved to recovery shortly. The nurse asks, "Have you spoken with the doctor yet?"

We're sitting and waiting for him to appear or for the phone to ring. The surgery sure seemed short from what they originally estimated. I'm not quite sure what to make of the shortened operation. Could it be that the arm needed to be amputated?

11:05: We just heard from Dr. Shives, and he got the tumor out with clean margins. They were able to save one of the nerves that they thought was in jeopardy. The tumor was 85 percent viable (alive). The pathologist will look at the tumor today and tomorrow, then Dr. Shives and Dr. Rodriguez, along with their group, will get together to discuss how to proceed. The main issue is recurrence. In the meantime, Hannah has the radiation tubes in place and her arm is vacuum sealed until Thursday.

Thank you for your continued prayers.

12:15: Hannah was wheeled back to the room from recovery. Waiting for her to come down the hallway seemed like two hours instead of the hour that it actually was from surgery to recovery to the room.

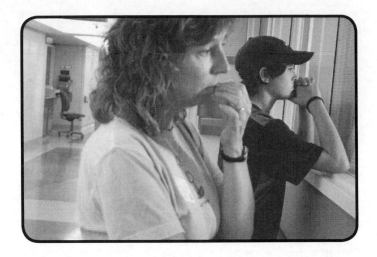

Sam and Kim wait outside the room as Hannah was lifted and shifted. The process is painful for her, but once she got settled in, she immediately went into resting mode.

The doctors will be around sometime later today or tonight to discuss the overall surgery. In the meantime, we're writing down questions to ask. Each room is conveniently set up with a white board and dry erase marker.

With her arm wrapped up to look twice its normal size, it had a look of an alien. The radiation tubes that projected over the top of her fingers from the end of the gauze and bandage, gave the appearance of long tentacles. These tubes will be used by Dr. Laack for radiation treatments. The nurse also did a little sensor nerve test on Hannah to see if she could identify all of her fingers being touched. Hannah was able to identify each one except for the pinkie finger, to which the ulnar nerve was connected and severed during surgery.

Currently we're waiting for the pump to be hooked up for her pain medication, but I suppose since she's asleep, all is good in the world of recovery.

"Later today, you're scheduled for a CT scan," the nurse tells us as she finishes adjusting Hannah's multiple tubes.

"For what?" Kim questions, since no one mentioned it before. We're then told that Dr. Laack probably wants to check the tubes in her arm. I, personally, can't imagine moving her again.

1:15: The pain pump is up and ready. Christine, our nurse, gave Hannah the rundown on the button and gave her specific instructions to not let Dad or brothers hit the button for her. So much for being able to watch ESPN when she finally comes around ... with one press of the button, the medicine would knock her out for another hour or so.

We're supposed to get her up and sitting as soon as she's able. It seems impossible right now. But hey, this whole cancer thing seems impossible from time-to-time.

2:30: The doctors stopped by and gave us the update. We are being shipped downtown by ambulance for the radiation CT by four today. Hannah's still pretty groggy so getting her up and moving is going to be a challenge.

The doctors also talked about the removal of her tumor and how its 85 percent viability makes them lean more toward amputation to prevent the higher percentage of recurrence. The pathologist's preliminary biopsy, taken from a small section of the tumor, was the showing the 85 percent. Dr. Shives did say that there have been a few cases where the main report came back with a lower percentage of viability, in which case they proceeded with the reconstruction. He did caution us that this is very unlikely.

The pathology report should be complete by tomorrow (hopefully, because some take up to thirty-six hours) and by late afternoon we will know. In the meantime, we continue forward with the radiation as planned for tomorrow.

3:45–8:30: We took the transport to the radiation center downtown. Hannah needed to have scans, simulations, and when all was set up and done, she received her first dose of radiation.

Dr. Laack and the radiology staff went into overtime to get Hannah's first radiation done. We even had the cleaning crew come and go while we waited. Tomorrow morning we'll take another ambulance ride back for all–day radiation. She'll receive three doses over the course of the day. The nice thing is that they will admit us into the Methodist Hospital (which is downtown) for the day, so we can go back to a room for more rest.

A Day in the Sun, or Just Radiation

Day 96:

Today is a big day as the doctors come together (after the final pathology report arrives) and discuss what will be the next step.

On one hand, we have Dr. Laack, who works with a great deal of adult sarcomas that behave similarly to Hannah's. They don't normally have a high percentage of the tumors being dead upon removal, yet with the same radiation Hannah is receiving, they have a 90 percent success rate of no recurrence.

On the other hand, we have Dr. Rodriguez, who works in childhood oncology. She had told us before that she was very uncomfortable with keeping the arm if the tumor still had life to it. If you amputate, you have a 100 percent chance that the tumor will not recur. However, even with amputation you still don't have a guarantee that the cancerous cells haven't already traveled to the lungs.

We're out of hands at this point, but we still have Dr. Shives, who has done extensive work with all kinds of sarcomas. He's the guy in the middle. From what I can read of Dr. Shives, he sees benefit along with risk in both cases. Yesterday, it seemed like he was leaning toward the 100 percent non–recurrence ... amputation.

There is a 20 to 30 percent chance that the cancer will spread to the lungs, no matter what. They just can't tell if micro–cancerous cells are present or not. This is the case with most cancers though. That's the reason Hannah will have scans every three months for a while. If the cells are present, then they would possibly show up over a three–month period or longer.

All of the doctors are waiting on the pathology report (although they don't think it will change much from the original read), talking with their respective groups here at Mayo and around the nation, and will be sitting down to present what they feel is the best possible move forward.

Late this afternoon we should know if tomorrow brings amputation or reconstruction.

6:30 a.m.: We were scheduled for another ambulance ride to downtown for radiation treatments. The one problem with this plan is that no one at the ambulance service was aware that they needed to take us.

7:30: The ambulance service has finally made it to pick up Hannah. Not a big deal, we are just about an hour off of our planned schedule today. It's not like we have to be somewhere else, so little glitches like this are no big deal.

9:00: We completed radiation, which was painful for Hannah since tape was used to hold some tubes in place. Apparently, when they went to remove the tape, it also moved the tubes inside her arm. The nerve is extremely sensitive after the surgery. We made it up to our new room at Methodist Hospital, where Hannah zonked out shortly after the nurses completed their initial check–in procedures. With the late start, we won't head back downstairs for more radiation until one this afternoon.

5:00: If you've been waiting for the time to jump up and down ... do it now!

Dr. Shin and Dr. Bishop just left the room. "It wasn't clear until twenty minutes ago, and now it makes a lot of sense. We will proceed with reconstruction," reported Dr. Shin.

The pathology report came in, the doctors did their research, and the consensus was to move ahead with the reconstruction.

Dr. Bishop also gave a bit of information that we hadn't heard before: "With the type of tumor she had, if it comes back, it is not likely to metastasize." This type of tumor just recurs in the same area, if at all. If this were to happen, then amputation would be the next step.

Kim questioned the doctors with, "Are you absolutely sure this is the right decision?" Without missing a beat, Dr. Shin responded, "We both have daughters, and if this were our daughter, we would do this procedure."

The surgery should take about four hours and will be first thing tomorrow morning.

A bonus bit of news from the doctors was that Hannah's thumb moved. This meant absolutely nothing to me because that's what I thought it was supposed to do, but then Dr. Shin explained how he had cut a nerve or tendon or something that goes to it to make the thumb move. Apparently she has some cross-wiring already occurring, thus making reconstruction even easier. Dr. Bishop did say that he would have to remove nerves from the bottom of both legs in order to build the graph.

What I didn't know was that even though the graph will be in place after tomorrow, it will only begin working at the rate of about one inch per month. So within seven to nine months, the nerve should be fully grown and feeling fine. Hannah will need further rehab and possible surgery in the future as the muscles and tendons adjust.

To You

It's amazing the number of people that write to us and express the way in which they have been touched and moved through our family and our experience.

From our view, everyone that has reached out on our behalf, prayed for Hannah, shared our story, are our heroes; you are our inspiration, you are our strength. We read in daily e-mails, comments, and cards about people who have lifted Hannah and our family up in prayer. We are overwhelmed, we are grateful, but most of all, we are blessed. It's a blessing to have such strong people behind us and in front of us, leading the prayer charge. You have not only stood strong in faith, but you have kept us just standing. We are so thankful to have such heroes in our lives.

Keep praying, keep reading.

Second Round

Day 97:
It's not even seven in the morning, and we've already had Pastor Kuddes stop by for a devotion and prayer. He's been a remarkable person in our lives. Each day, he's come to the hospital to visit with us and to pray with our family.

We also had a visit from Dr. Neeley, who works with Dr. Shives. He stopped by to let us know that although they were taking a backseat to Dr. Shin's and Dr. Bishop's services, they were still following along. And that's why we're here—the team concept.

6:45: Blood work is done. We're ready for surgery. Hannah's a bit more nervous today. With surgery on her legs, she knows that the pain will be a bit more than on Tuesday.

8:15: Today's procedure is supposed to be around four hours. I once again donned the blue bunny suit for the walk back to the operating room with Hannah. The operating teams are probably happy to get rid of me because I like to ask a lot of questions—there are just too many cool machines. Since Hannah had the IV already in place, she didn't need the mask. The doctor gave one plunge of the milky–white fluid, and Hannah closed her eyes. "Can you open your eyes for us?" asked the nurse. Nothing—she was out. Just that quick.

The procedure to have a tendon transfer, take nerves from both legs, and tie up the loose ends has started. We wait in the lobby, staring at the monitor which displays progress in the operating room. "Procedure started," reads the flat screen.

12:30: We just left the doctors; Hannah has had a successful surgery. They opened her arm up just above the elbow in order to move the ulnar nerve and gain more length. The nerve runs on the backside of the elbow, so they just moved it to the inside (gaining centimeters).

They also completed the tendon transfer. If you were to take your palm and face it down, flex your wrist. There are a few tendons in there that allow flexing. They were able to take one out (now turn your wrist over) and place it on the pinkie side of her arm to help with finger flexing.

Hannah will be sore where her legs were opened up (lower calves) in order to get the nerves, but she should be able to get up and move. I'm going to bet that she won't want to move. She will also have a hard shell that will go from just above her elbow, down her arm, and around the topside of her hand (so her hand will remain bent and not stretch the tendons). In three weeks, she should be able to be taken out of that.

Peace and prayers.

So Many Tubes

Day 97 (post surgery):
Getting through the pain.

It's been a long afternoon of painful shifting of pillows and of Hannah. With every movement came a bit of discomfort, some more painful than others. Who would have thought that putting a pillow under her legs would cause severe pain, but after we did it, the tears streaming down her face were an indication.

Hannah has a pain threshold that rebounds quickly. She will yell and cry when it hurts, but within minutes of moving her, she rebounds and the pain is gone.

The nurses have told her that she need not move through recovery in one night. She wants to be up. She wants to be disconnected from all the wires and tubes. She wants to be able to stretch and scratch an itch when it occurs, all when she just needs to rest.

High School Musical 2 is on tomorrow evening (along with a new *Hannah Montana*), so you know we'll be pushing through recovery in preparation.

Just Keep Moving

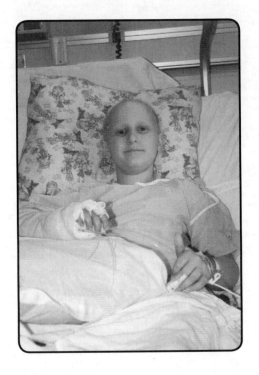

Day 98:
I can't help but think of *Finding Nemo* with Dory *(just keep swimming, just keep swimming)* when it comes to Hannah's nurse. The goal for today is movement.

Hannah began this morning with being unable to bend her feet up toward her body. She's since been up and down trying to walk. Who would have thought that something that seems so simple can become so difficult?

Her legs have bandages on them because of her allergy to tape. The doctors decided the best option would be to wrap rather than tape. Hannah has two incisions (right down the middle) running from the back of her lower legs to just below her knees. Dr. Bishop explained that they would put it right in the middle so that when she wears stockings, the scar will be covered. I couldn't help but think, *Stockings? She's ten.* I suppose it makes sense for later though.

Alli stopped by to visit with Hannah before she left for home today. Alli has leukemia and runs back and forth to Mayo for treatments. She, too, is a ten-year-old, blond-haired girl who was actually growing her hair long for Locks of Love when she was diagnosed. We first met her and her mom at the House. Alli will be starting radiation soon, so Hannah gets to be the guide and share the experience with her. It's always a sharing time when it comes to kids with cancer around the RMH.

Time for more walking. We're going to try and make it to the door this time. Usually it takes Kim on the arm side to hold the pillow, me taking a side for support, and then the nurse or a grandma handling the poll and tubes … and, oh yeah, Hannah has the middle.

Please send prayers for healing and strength in walking. Hannah has also been spiking a fever off and on.

Peace and prayers.

Running Ahead

Day 99:

The last day of the double digit, and it was prayers answered once again. Yesterday I left a little girl in a great deal of pain, who was having difficulty walking around the end of her bed, and with a person on each side of her with a poll in tow.

This morning I walked into the room to find her exiting the bathroom, smile on her face, no poll, no bandages, and only the help of mom holding a pillow under her right arm.

I instantly recalled the night after her first surgery. We were tired, frustrated, and living in the unknown of what was to come. I left the hospital that evening and headed back to the House. While I walked, I had one of those private–public chats with God. "You are the only one that can bring a miracle here." The next day we received the news that she was moving forward with reconstruction. Then as they examined her, a thumb twitched that shouldn't have been possible after the Tuesday surgery. Step by step we see prayers being answered. This morning, she walked.

The back of her legs were covered with what the doctors referred to as "big Band–Aids." They were much better than her wraps with the bonus of scratch–ability.

The doctors informed us that Hannah should be discharged some time tomorrow. By being removed from all drips, lines, and hookups, along with her ability to walk, she has made enough progress to get out of the hospital and continue her recovery back in our room at the Ronald McDonald House.

The good thing is if anything were to go south, the hospital is two blocks away. To celebrate the milestone in her recovery, we broke out the snow cone maker (Hucke–style) and proceeded with the brain freeze.

Speaking of the Huckes, Dawn and Danielle stopped by on their way out of town, while Hannah and Max were having a little Webkinz time. It was a nice moment to share with others who had just been down our road. We have some recovery ahead, as well as some concerns that still remain. Talking and sharing is a wonderful outlet.

We've had several talks with the various groups of doctors. The latest have been about that Hannah has a 40 percent chance of the cancer spreading (regardless of what's been done). Just when we thought we were put through it, we're now told that she is still at risk—a 40 percent risk. Talk about swallowing deep.

We can choose to worry or we can choose to trust. With what has already taken place, I know that prayers are being heard. It's hard not to slip once in a while to that dark side of thought, but when we remember to stay in the light, we have great days; and it's all about cherishing the time you have.

Evacuee is the Name

Day 100:

You would think that on the one hundredth day we might be surprised with a little Zero the Hero (a fictional character used in elementary schools to celebrate the one hundredth day of school) running to and fro, or at least pictures of my friend Gary in tights and a cape running around his house. Oh no! At around five a.m., we got the, "Your attention please, the Ronald McDonald House is under an evacuation. Please gather the necessary items and prepare to leave immediately."

It came through the phone system, which was a lot like the hospital intercom system, so the two blended nicely into my delirious state of snooze. As I snapped out of it, I realized where I was, which was not at the hospital.

Are you serious? Did she say evacuation?

As I stumbled from the bed to the phone to call the front desk, the words kept resonating in my head—followed quickly with thoughts of *there's no way this is possibly happening.*

"We are under an immediate evacuation. The fire department has authorized the evacuation and is here to assist. Gather as much as you can, but you need to go immediately," came the voice once again, as if I weren't paying attention the first time.

Yep, it's happening.

Again with the word *immediately*. Are they not aware that it's just the boys and me and no concept of adequate packing skills? Leaving it up to us to determine what's important and what's not is not a good idea. After assessing the room, I was sure about one item that needed to go for sure—my new *Wild Hogs* DVD (bikers out there know what I'm thinking).

I also made the phone call to Kim at the hospital. "Can you come to the House for a moment?" That wasn't well received since she had Hannah to think of and it was five in the morning.

Onto the next call. My parents were in town for the surgery and were about ten minutes away from the Ronald McDonald House. "Come quick, we're being evacuated!" I spent little time explaining my confusion about the whole phone evacuation warning.

It had been raining extremely hard all day yesterday and throughout the night. Unfortunately, RMH sits at the bottom of a rather large hill, which put us in a mudslide zone. Apparently, the evacuee grapevine had mud breaking through a retaining wall and flooding into one room on the first floor, falling power lines, and trees being uprooted. I was trying to decide which pillows were ours and which ones belonged to the House.

Needless to say, evacuation procedures will be added to the résumé. We got almost everything out before the firemen told us that we only needed a couple of days' worth of stuff because they would most likely have everything under control by then. That's comforting to know, and I can now stop my FEMA process of evacuation.

I later told Kim and Hannah of our heroism— how we faced mud and didn't flinch; how we managed the complex move of one American Girl Doll, a wig, and many other valuable items too numerous to mention. I'm sure the professional firemen were overly impressed by the amount of stuff we had gathered over the months and managed to jam into two cars.

Hannah gets released from the hospital tomorrow. Fortunately, the Huckes are on vacation this week and have offered their home as a getaway if we need a break. I would say this qualifies as a getaway.

101 Is Not a Radio Station

Day 102:
Seeking refuge in Byron (west of Rochester) at the Hucke getaway, we've settled into a "Fluffy" way of life. Fluffy is one of the Hucke's cats. Fluffy seems to have the attitude of staying cool while being laid back. When Hannah was released from the hospital, she made fast action in calling the big, leather chair right away and began her Fluffy training.

Things are going well as we wait for the Ronald McDonald House to get back to operating order. I stopped by today and picked up an *Anytime* coupon to McDonalds. As long as we are out of the House, we can go to any Rochester area McDonalds and receive free food. If only I hadn't seen that movie *Super Size Me*. It is really putting a damper on a good thing. We haven't told Max just yet, but it will be like winning the lotto for him.

Late night is always the right time for a trip to the emergency room. Hannah spiked a fever and once we hit the 101 mark, it's a road trip. Blood work and other samples taken, the doctors and nurses are working on a cause. They even placed a call to the surgical service team to have her arm uncovered and looked at for any possible infections.

It's just past one fifteen in the morning, and we're settling into our new room. It seems like we just left this place yesterday—wait, we did.

The doctors want to watch Hannah without antibiotics overnight to see if they can narrow down the source of the infection. I'm not quite sure if this will be good in terms of a good night's sleep, but I'm guessing that as soon as I finish writing, it won't take long to fall sleep.

Every Day, Something New

Day 103:

After 103 days, we are still learning new things.

Dr. Shin and his team stopped by this morning to review our nightly endeavors. Actually, to my disbelief, rounds began at six thirty this morning. That makes a total of six hours of sleep for me in two days. They say that your brain turns to mush if you don't get enough sleep. In my case, I've passed mush and moved right into liquid goo.

It seems that there are two types of temperatures. One is the not normal (above the 98.6), then there's the surgical temperature. Hannah's temperature from last night wasn't close to the surgical temperature. In other words, *keep the bandage on, avoid exposure, and "Why wasn't I called?"*

The wound was open, and that's what we have to face today. As for infection, the area that the doctors felt might have been infected was actually red due to the radiation. Dr. Shin was well aware that the skin would have a higher rate of recovery and that the redness was a cause, not a concern.

We ended up in the cast room, where Hannah was once again exposed and readied for the next step: casting. The need to keep her arm immobile over the next three weeks is key to allowing the tendons to recover.

Cool side note: I was allowed to see the reconstruction photos today (Kim opted not to look, for reasons of nausea). They were unbelievable in the way they showed the transfer of nerves and tendons. The photo of the tumor itself was surreal to look at. It was just over two inches in width by almost five inches in length, and it even seemed to have an evil look to it. If I knew it wouldn't have seemed weird or landed me in psychological treatment, I probably would have yelled a few foul words at it. There must have been at least twenty pictures to the staging and all were fascinating to see.

In the casting room, we had the talented Nurse Tracey (the resident "feel good" nurse). She not only found the purple casting material to brighten the smile on Hannah's face, but she also added a little artistic flair with flowers and hearts. Just when we thought it was all done, the glitter glue came out and the smear was on! Hannah's cast is on and looking sparkly in the sun.

Prayers for zero metastasizing cells along with healthy checkups in the next two weeks. Our next step is to hear from the oncology group on Monday, with chemotherapy to begin on the thirty–first.

Keep reading, keep praying.

Saying Good-bye to Michigan

Day 104:

It's great to say hello to friends you haven't seen in a while, but it's something quite different when it comes to saying goodbye. We had to do it three times within a twenty-four-hour period.

It seems that when people journey west to Mayo, they tend to do it at or around the same time, and when they leave, it's an exodus. This past week we had the Hs: Hosbein and Husmann. They are two wonderful families from Michigan who came to do the Mayo thing. The Mayo thing, as I'm finding out, is one of those bonding experiences, like joining a club—only there's no secret handshake, we just say a lot of prayers together and for one another.

Our time hasn't been exceptionally freeing for visiting. Yet, despite the land of medical procedures and appointments, we did manage some time.

Beach Gary and Barb had been kept busy by their own doctors, but the short amount of time we had was well spent and really meant more than I could begin to tell them. As for the Husmann group, it was feed bag and visiting time as we took down a local buffet dining house before they had to leave for Michigan. Both of these families are fighting for a healthier tomorrow as they trek back and forth from Michigan to Mayo. Both families know exactly what we are going through when it comes to living in a Mayo world. It's prayers, doctors, nurses, and families joined together.

The toughest goodbye was the one closest to the heart—the boys were going home (with Grandma and Grandpa) to prepare for the start of school. Max was the toughest. Not that saying goodbye to Sam was easier (he hugged me, for the record), but Sam understands that our time of separation is necessary.

After our spring separation, when we came home after being gone for weeks, I bent down and wrapped Max up in my arms and told him, "We will never be apart again. I promise."

Those very words came back to me late last night as Max reminded me of a dad's promise. How could I not keep my promise? It was tough to look into his tear–filled eyes and tell him that I had to break that promise.

Kim and I toiled all night. Do we put emphasis on education or emotional balance? We had talked it out to the point where we were ready to give up the beginning of school and keep him when he strolled slowly into bedroom, sad face and all, sat on the bed next to us and said, "I'll let you decide." That was our emotional okay to send him home (although still not the easiest thing to do).

So if you see Max, give him a hug from us and remind him we'll be home soon. You could even give Sam one too, even though he'll never admit that he likes a hug every now and then (thirteen–year–olds, go figure). Also remind them that although saying good-bye may be hard, we will get back to the other side of that spectrum very soon and be on our way back to Michigan.

This Monday we have an oncology appointment to discuss pathology, decisions that were made, and what we do from this point (besides more chemotherapy).

Peace and prayers.

Just Like Earnhardt

Day 105:

After a rousing morning of Madden 2007 (PlayStation 2 game), I'm happy to report that the Bears are in the Super Bowl. Let the shuffle begin again.

The afternoon brought about practice and game planning for my Monsters of the Midway in digital form. It also brought about a phone call from the Decker family.

Who doesn't remember Shanna, the cancer dancer girl? If you don't remember, simply refer to the "Girl Time," entry to refresh yourself. And like most of us in the society of childhood cancer who are often referred to as "the parents of ... ," there's Shanna's mom, Sherrie, and Shanna's dad, Jack.

We had the pleasure of spending an evening of grill time (not to be confused with girl time because Jack and I were present) and conversation with them. The awesomeness of sharing this one–on–one time is that we once again had the chance to talk with those who have been down that road and continue to be there. It's still one of those things that I sit back and find myself trying to take in because it is so new.

After dinner we took a walk to the Wabasha Implement Company (owned and operated by the Deckers), where Hannah and Shanna took to the zero–radius mowing mammoth of NASCAR out for a little round about.

The smiles on their faces said it all as they went in circles like the tops of old. Hannah operated one handle while Shanna worked the other. Two working as one; a team is formed. Just like in treatments, we rely on others to help us through. These two girls understand that more clearly than most and took to it naturally.

Then came my turn on the machine. *Instruction? I don't need instruction. I've seen Stripes, Hogans Heroes, Caddy Shack… okay, maybe just a little instruction.* Shanna gave me the basics, and I was off like Earnhardt pulling into the pit after a flat tire, engine on fire, and fiberglass clinging to its last remaining piece of duct tape. The only thing that was missing on my ride was a set of stick–on flames on the side panel. The machine was smooth. It handled me better than I it. I had a flashback to my first childhood mowing experience when I couldn't decide which side of the new sapling I would choose—so I ran over it. There, another childhood secret out. See what zero radius does to me?

The walk home wouldn't have been complete without a little help from a friend, as Shanna carries Hannah's pillow so she can get her arm up and give it a rest from the cast.

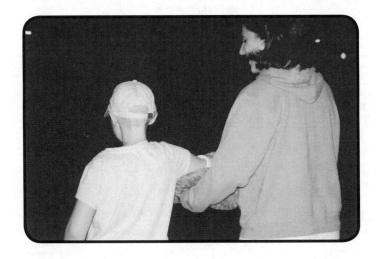

Super Bowl Sunday tomorrow—I need to get some sleep.

Peace and prayers.

Decker Day

Day 106:

As of this moment, the Super Bowl has been postponed—save the shuffle for midweek (what else do you have to do in the middle of work week?).

Today we traveled back to Plainview for some more Deckertime. Shanna had mentioned her lack of Harley time the night before, and when you couple that with a church service on a Sunday morning, you have the makings of a good start to your day.

I felt more at home on two wheels than I had on that scooter–mower–donut–maker, so I knew it was my turn to return the favor of instruction. *Today was the day to make Shanna a Harley chick!*

If you ever find your travels taking you to Minnesota, a *must view* would be the area of Lake Pepin. The view from the bike was spectacular as we cruised the Mississippi. I'm almost positive that Shanna found the experience to be fantastic!

As visitors in Lake City, we decided to take a little cruise on a paddleboat. The girls couldn't wait to see what the action on the boat looked like as they peered through the window, hoping not to find that disgruntled employee from *Scooby–Doo* who always chased away the kids.

Hannah did a little walking of the plank before our boarding call. Part of Hannah's therapy—when it came to her legs—is to get in a great deal of walking.

The more walking she can manage, the faster the healing process. Shanna kept her walking as they strolled back and forth on the dock.

While on our three–hour cruise on the *SS Minnow*, we had more time to share relaxing times, good company, and Hannah attempting the one–arm tying of a bow (at which she eventually succeeded).

One of the more fascinating bits of information we were made privy to was the building of a Viking ship on the shores of Wisconsin. Yep, all you cheese lovers heard me correctly. The story is going to be covered nationally. They are building a Viking ship on cheese soil. Now, here's where the story takes a twist.

It seems that once the construction (which begins in early September) is concluded, the ship is to be set ablaze (big flames and smoke). I don't know if this strikes anyone else as "taunting" the other side, but this is on the eve of the NFL revving up, and I'm just not sure of the impression that's being given. What I am sure of is that some big–name columnist will have an easy time writing this story and that the tickets will be sold out for the Vikings–Packers game.

One more thing before I go. Happy birthday, Shanna (this Tuesday). Hope the surprise party works out— although I know nothing about it, so I know there's no Harley ride planned. Plus, happy birthday to Sherrie (that's Shanna's mom, in case you missed it earlier). I'm sure Shanna has your surprise party well in hand.

Rounding Third and Heading for Home

Day 107:

Incredible. Shocking. Surreal.

We had late meetings today with Dr. Rodriguez, Dr. Shives, and Dr. Laack. It was as if they were taking numbers outside the room where we sat. As one would finish, another would enter to chat with us.

Dr. Rodriguez was first with the chemotherapy and long–term effects. It seems that while studies won't be conclusive for another ten to twelve years out, they can't be sure if chemotherapy is a help or hindrance. While it could possibly be killing any microscopic cancer cells floating around, it also has the possibility of bringing on future cancers. *Great, a double–edged sword.* We will have three more chemo treatments to go, starting in September.

Dr. Laack was next. *What could she be telling us? Her part is done—a shot of radiation and it's done.* Actually, Dr. Laack is a whole lot more than that. She spent time at an oncology seminar where Hannah seemed to be the patient of topic. Her tumor was one that was puzzling a number of doctors. Dr. Laack explained to us that her first tumor (diagnosed as fibromatosis—not cancerous), could have possibly been misdiagnosed and that she really had what they call NSFP. There's a longer name for it, but quite honestly she lost me at *misdiagnosis.*

It's one of those things that you can look back at and ask why they didn't catch it, or you put your faith in check and understand that this path has already been laid out.

It seems that Mayo, in the last two years, has had the leading pathologist in sarcomas join the staff. He took one look at the slides from her 1998 biopsy and said it was this tumor, which starts off benign and over time has the tendency to change to a malignancy. Dr. Laack asked us if her first tumor ever had a discoloration on the surface of the skin.

"Well, yes. It had a reddish color to it," we responded as if she had just done a reading from a crystal ball.

"That's one of the telltale signs to this type of cancers," she said with the certainty of Columbus finding the new world. Actually, it's a lot like that. You sail around cancer for a while until you spot land, or in our case, the tumor with which we are dealing. And, just like Columbus discovering India, Dr. Laack tells us that this isn't 100 percent for sure—but it's pretty close.

The reason that no one knew about the discoloration before is because we had the first tumor biopsied in Chicago and then moved over to Mayo. The scar had covered the discoloration.

The tumor she described is slow growing, which is good because the percentages change. Instead of a 40 percent chance of it spreading to the lungs, we now look at a 10 to 15 percent chance. The rate of recurrence is around the one–to–two–year period. If it's coming back, that's the mark that they look at. You see, in the cancer world, it's all about time and percentages.

The third to see us was Dr. Shives. He explained the procedure of tumor removal and what clean margins mean when it comes to microscopic cells. In short, not a whole lot. With a tumor like Hannah's, it's almost impossible to get a completely clear field. The tumor was resting on nerves and muscles, but that's why Dr. Laack went in the night of surgery and began her radiation treatment.

The last words we heard from each member of the staff overseeing Hannah's case was, "Go home."

What? If they're talking about the Ronald McDonald House, we can't because it's still closed. But they weren't talking about good 'ole RMH.

"Go home. Chemotherapy doesn't start until next Thursday, and you have no other appointments until then. Go home."

I don't think I've seen a bigger smile on Hannah's face in quite a while. Even while Dr. Laack talked with Kim, Hannah kept looking at me and mouthing the word *home* with this wonderful ear–to–ear grin. I must admit, it did bring that untouchable tingle down my back as well. Part of it was because it means I get to ride my Harley for an entire day as we travel back to

Michigan, and the other part was, well, you can probably guess.

We've met such wonderful families since we've been here. Like Kim said, "I feel like I'm leaving home all over again." That says a lot for all the families that have touched our lives. When you have such a connection, it is hard to wrap your head around it. We had to pack a van full of months of living, make calls to tell everyone in the Sota that we were leaving for Michigan, and I still don't think I got to everyone. Those that we did contact gathered briefly at Buffalo Wild Wings for a "see you soon, happy you're going" style party. With Hannah's treatments, we will be back for chemotherapy three more times, plus scans every two months.

Taking One Pile at a Time

Day 110:
It was great to get back to our home after a three month stint ... and it was not so great. The thing about being gone for so long is that you have things to do *or to repair* when you get back.

"The toilet handle is droopy!" *What?*

"The hot water isn't working right!" *Huh?*

"The back of the dryer had the tube just blow off and sent lint all over!" *Oh, sweet Nelly!*

Coming home has the feeling of my year spent in pony league baseball. My coach used to drop us off at home. By drop us off, I mean literally. He would slow down enough for you to make a jump for it from the back of his pickup, giving weight to the phrase "hit the ground running." This feels similar, only I haven't given up all hope and tucked into a ball for rolling purposes…just yet.

Anyone who's been gone for a period of time can relate to the amount of stuff that you can accumulate. For those who never had the experience, go to your basement or attic, pack everything up, haul it outside and place it in the back of your car, drive around for a while talking about how you can't see out the back window, and then bring it all home again for unpacking. I have this plastic tub at the foot of my bed (since I've been back to work) that acts as a footlocker. Little by little, we work through it by taking it one pile at a time. I just hope nobody needs anything quickly.

The upside is a terrific guy named Steve (a fellow teacher) has mowed the yard. I'm checking it off my list and moving on to another pile! It's the little things like what Steve did that makes me appreciate others so much.

Hannah has gone to school twice so far and loves it. She was a bit sad to not be with her friends playing basketball, but just like the droopy toilet handle, things will pick up.

September

Hello, Livery

Day 115:
It's Mug Club Night. For most that means nothing, for others, those three words say it all.

The Livery is a wonderful microbrewery located in downtown Benton Harbor. Over one hundred years ago it was known as a gathering place called the Palace Livery. It has been resurrected and once again become a gathering place for local residents as well as for travelers passing through. I haven't heard anyone yell "Norm!" just yet, but I do get a first name greeting when I walk through the door.

Being home has been a bit more than a day's adjustment. Our piles at home turned into major reorganization projects—although I really didn't get to downsize anything. The school load is getting under some control. It's different being back. While Kim and I are treading water trying to wrap our minds around everyday stuff, you can't help but be in a different place than others around you. Our time out of our normal lives has somehow altered what normal is to us.

It's tough to switch gears and think *normal*. As we prepare to head back to Mayo, we have been trying to balance the two lives. It's hard to explain, but the two just don't mesh yet. What I used to find important, I now find minimal in the grand scheme of things; so it takes actually more effort for me to put my whole heart and soul into it, for example, setting up bulletin boards in my classroom.

In the meantime, we are able to reconnect with friends and family, which is the most important part when it comes to support and being home.

We are heading back to Mayo on Wednesday. Hannah has tests early Thursday, the cast comes off, and chemotherapy begins again.

See you in Minnesota, you betcha! I hope someone has a hot dish waiting for us when we get in.

Using Big Words Just Means You've Been Around Too Long

Day 116:
Back at the Ronald McDonald House, which just reopened, we settle into our fourth room. I don't know

if I can say that one room is that much different from the other, and I definitely don't want to use the words "it feels like home," but I will go as far as to say it feels comfortably familiar.

Hannah settles into her bottom bunk as we prepare for a big day tomorrow. We begin with an echocardiogram (which takes about one to two hours) first thing in the morning to make sure that her heart is able to withstand the chemotherapy treatment. Then we head off for a venipuncture specimen collection (blood test). Just when we think we've had enough testing for the morning, we still need to get an electrocardiogram, which records the electrical activity of the heart. All of this information will be forwarded to our oncologist, Dr. Rodriguez, for an afternoon appointment before admitting Hannah to the hospital for chemotherapy. Just in case we find free time, we're supposed to see Dr. Shin for a cast removal and stitches tomorrow. Who needs to work on a diet when you have the Mayo schedule?

There is something special about being back in Minnesota. We're back with the wonderful friends that we've had the pleasure of getting to know this summer. It is just something indescribable when a true connection develops with people whom you just met over a summer; and they care for your family as if they've known you forever. It's because of those connections that you know God is at work. We feel it daily from those who have reached out. Our family may be going down a road that most would dread, but it's a walk that has made us stronger and blesses us in ways that we could never have imagined. And yes, we pray daily that the message God wants us to learn has gotten through—now just make the cancer go away. We'll keep the friends and give back the cancer. It's a deal.

We also are back in the comfort zone of care. You develop a security blanket at the Mayo Clinic. I don't know how it happened or even when, but it does. The further you get, the less secure you feel and vice versa.

Prayer request: Testing goes well to start chemotherapy; strength through chemotherapy; appetite to keep weight up; Dr. Shin finds good results from his (and Dr. Bishop's) reconstruction; a safe return home early next week.

Peace and prayers.

Round Five Begins

Day 117:
It began like most days. "Could you shut the light off? I'm not ready to get up just yet!"

Whoever came up with the idea of a Sleep Number Bed is probably sleeping on a regular mattress in a really, really big house (laughing that he got people to purchase expensive beds that involve the same material used by small children in pools everywhere: the floatation wrap–around duck, which consists of air and plastic–sealed wrap). He and his brother (the guy who came up with selling water—that you can get for free—in a plastic bottle) must have great fun at our expense.

Take it from a Sleep Number veteran—unless you have a tent over the top of you and the ground inches below, never put an air mattress in your home. There, I said it. Now let's hear from those air–mattress people who sleep on clouds.

We made our way downtown for the series of tests, which went exceptionally well as we bounced from waiting room to exam room to another waiting room and so on. Hannah was cleared to begin chemotherapy tonight and the killing of any micro–cancer cells that may be left. The sooner the better I say!

Hannah was a bit nervous about getting back to the chemo routine. After all, it's been since the end of July when we finished the fourth treatment. Her hair is coming back (baby soft), her energy is up, and now we shoot her full of the drugs that will basically take her to ground zero. Of course, she's a bit apprehensive.

The nice thing is that since being back at Mayo, our support group has responded already. We had dinner with Pastor Kuddes and Naomi, his daughter, we heard from the Deckers, we're hooking up with the Hucke family tomorrow, and when checking into the hospital today, our nurse was Julia (we like Julia a lot).

The icing on the cake was when we walked down the hall, after a brief break from the hospital earlier in the evening, to find Amber as the charge nurse.

We are seriously thinking about completing our last two chemotherapy treatments back in Michigan, but it's people like these that make a decision like this a tough one. Our hope is to have our two worlds (of friends and family) meet someday.

Prayers: Strength through chemo and that it does the job on any micro–cells that may be left.

Upon Your Return

Day 118:
The calm before the storm.

Rolling out of bed this morning at the House, I thought to myself, *this is the day we peel back the cast, remove the stitches, and see what came from the reconstruction.*

Upon my return to the hospital, Sarah, the child life specialist, informed us that the U.S. Navy was paying a visit to the hospital and that we could meet them in the atrium. Being an Air Force guy, I felt that the Navy was close enough (they fly planes, too), so I had no qualms. The coffee cup went on the counter and off we went (not into the wild blue yonder, just down the hallway).

Hannah had a number of Navy guys to talk to, and they did a wonderful job at making her feel at ease. I was probably more interested when it came to comparing the two branches of service. We heard everything from ships to subs. They even gave Hannah a few Navy keepsakes before they departed.

After a brief meeting with the Navy, we decided to ease into the rest day. We finally began to see the doctors on rounds. Well, almost see the doctors. We decided to make a run to the hospital library to see what interesting tales from Hollywood sat on the shelves (a little in–room movie was on our minds for the afternoon).

Upon returning to the room, Bethany (our nurse) informed us that we just missed the doctors, but not to worry because they would be back. *So close to finding out about the cast, stitches, future treatments, and schedules!*

Dr. Arndt (who was an officer in the Navy) was on rounds today. If you were to ask anyone at Mayo about Dr. Arndt, I believe the word *guru* would pop up in several descriptions. She explained that Hannah would be perfectly fine receiving chemotherapy back in Michigan and that scans would more than likely be determined as we got closer. Just as she wrapped up, Dr. Shin's and Dr. Bishop's resident came in to see us. He put together orders to have the cast removed on Monday. *Monday? What about physical therapy? What about stitches? What about us going home?*

"Dr. Bishop is scheduled for rounds tomorrow," he told us as if passing decisions on to the main guy. "I've just set up a temporary plan."

We thought, *that's it then.* The rest of the day we'll spend watching movies and soaking up the chemo. Not so fast! Hannah had a hunger for an ice cream bar, which they had in the main floor cafeteria. Off I went like a man on a mission. I might not be able to do a number of things in a hospital, but finding an ice cream bar was a definite "can do" situation.

Upon my return to the room with dripping goodness in hand, I found our resident with a saw. Orders had been changed and the stitches and cast were coming off today, and the hand–therapy people were on their way.

Everything up to this point would have been considered the calm.

The removal of the cast took about an hour. It was excruciating with a lot of crying and screaming (mostly just me). The blade to make the first cut on the back of the arm was fine, but when the arm was turned over and the blade was right over the stitches, it was unbearable. So a new plan had to be thought through and more cuts made.

Then, to make matters worse, the tool which spreads the cast was rather large—apparently made for use on leg casts, although I thought a cast was a cast was a cast.

That's why the ice cream thing is up my alley. As the spreader was jammed repeatedly into the gap that was obviously too small, more and more jamming and pressing didn't seem to help much. Another plan was developed to make the cut in the cast larger. Did I mention it took about an hour? Bethany, our nurse, came in to help Hannah get through this cast removal, as well as to give pointers to the resident, who seemed to be working himself into a sweat. He was trying to peel the cast off of an arm that was stitched from wrist to elbow and extremely sensitive, and was doing it with all the wrong tools.

Eventually the cast was off! Next step was for the stitches to be removed.

Hannah knew it would hurt before he even took the scissors and tweezers out of the bag. The first few pull and snips were met with "ouch!" The resident was starting with the stitches on the topside of her hand, where the tendon had been cut for use on the other side of her wrist.

Oh, this is not going to go well. I looked at the other side of her arm laced with stitch after stitch, from wrist to elbow, spanning eight inches or so. With several breaks, wiping of tears, and deep breaths, we finally made it through the removal of all the stitches. As the stitches were being removed, it looked like they pulled the skin away from the arm, which didn't look quite healed and even began to bleed a little from some spots.

Dr. Shin had told us that with radiation, the wounds don't heal as fast. I also thought that this would be a concern for chemo since the arm needs to heal, and now it's losing all its strength to fight off anything, let alone heal. To the medical staff, everything looked great. I'm interested to hear what Dr. Bishop thinks on rounds tomorrow.

Following a half an hour or so of stitch removal, the hand specialists finally got to work on a little therapy and making a splint for Hannah. They did an excellent job working with Hannah, who was in a lot of pain already and had just about reached her limit of people working on her arm. The splint she received will have to be worn at all times to keep the tendons from stretching more than needed.

While Hannah picked purple for the splint because it's one of her favorite colors, others believe she picked it for the Vikings (sorry, Mrs. Swim. No Packer colors were offered).

After the extensive work, Hannah settled in for a late afternoon nap with her in–room movie playing.

We had dinner catered in by the Hucke family tonight. I knew Hannah was doing better when I asked her what she wanted for dinner. She replied, "Wings!"

Prayers for: Healthy recovery of her arm; chemo-therapy strength; the killing of all micro–cancer cells.

Peace and prayers.

For the Road

Day 120:

"Are you doing good this morning?" I thought it was safe question as I entered the room.

"I threw up," was Hannah's matter–of–fact reply.

Okay, so maybe we'll just hear about yesterday.

Bob and Lois, my newfound riding partners from Waltham Trinity Lutheran, had laid out Saturday plans. Besides it being their anniversary, there was a bike ride scheduled for the day. Bob had stopped by the hospital on Friday to visit and ever so casually mentioned the ride—and the fact that I could ride their Sportster. *Hmm, let me think about this for a min—okay!*

The ride left from the establishment Cheers in Waltham. While I didn't hear a great number of people yelling "Norm," rest assured that this was a place where everyone knew your name. The people on the ride were some of the nicest people you would want to meet. Guys like Johnny and Donny, along with Bob, Lois, and the crew, made me feel like I had been a part of the group for years. I just may have to bring my bike out on every trip to the "Land of a Thousand Lakes" (Bob pointed out a water treatment plant on the ride), just in case another ride springs up—or Shanna needs more lessons on things like "how to properly scream while discharging a bug from your mouth."

The ride was a planned benefit for cancer which made it even more personal for me. I even received a Cowbag shirt from the owners at the end of the ride. Cowbag is short for Cheers of Waltham Bar and Grill.

While I was out on the road, Hannah and Kim had the Deckers drop by for the evening. With *High School Musical 2* in hand, the girls enjoyed a little song-bird practice. I thought I felt a tingle down my spine while I was out riding—it was because I was missing the duet.

I also returned to find that Shanna had donated some of her hair in the name of good medicine.

Off to the playroom for a little Doctor Hannah examination.

One of Hannah's favorite things to do in the play-room is to play "medical examiner," which means, if you're in the hot seat, prepare for the once-over. Shanna apparently wasn't thinking clearly when she allowed Hannah to strap tape to her arm. One smooth motion and *rip,* the bandage is off, along with any hair you might have had. *Good gracious Maggie May, that had to hurt!* Hannah's either going into medicine, or she'll make a terrific waxer.

With Hannah feeling a little less well today, we're planning on hanging out in the hospital for a while, or until Bethany leaves. Bethany has been right by Han-nah's side on this trip. (Another reason why making the trip to Mayo is well worth it.) The fifth round is done, which leaves us just around seventeen days before we need to be back to do it all over again.

The orthopedic surgeons want to see Hannah in three weeks to see how her motion is progressing, so our plans on staying home for treatments in Michigan have been negated. In the meantime, Hannah has to wear a splint twenty–four hours a day. She doesn't have to wear a sling though, unless in crowded areas (like the school hallway), and that's just to keep her arm close to her body so it doesn't accidentally get bumped. Thanks for your prayers.

Keep reading, keep praying.

Holding Our Breath

Day 122:
Hannah's been home this week. A number of her classmates are out with varying illnesses. It's not a really good time to send her to school when her counts are on their way down.

She's also been battling a cough and has been oozing from her arm, although it's becoming less and less each day. Monday, right before leaving Rochester, she had her hand therapy with Cara, only to have the surgical service (aka: Matt the resident) pay her a visit. He went the safe route and placed her on an antibiotic.

It's as if we're waiting for the other shoe to drop as we hold our breath each day, praying for no infection.

Thursday is the official blood count day. Although it seems like this should be old hat at this point in the treatment, it never fails that something new enters the picture (this time it's her arm recovery).

As Hannah kicks back on the couch this week with homework, Kim and I are working back into the daily routine—not the easiest thing to do with so much on our minds.

Thank you for your prayers. They mean a great deal to us.

Peace and prayers.

Getting It Right

Day 124:

If it's a matter of the moment, then the question should be, "Does this moment matter?"

Being back in the midst of my classroom, I find myself engulfed by parental concerns, student struggles, and general educational issues. I actually got up this morning to be in school two hours early to work on school improvement before the doors swung open wide. Being a chairperson for the group, I want to take care of my responsibilities, and suddenly I'm finding myself concerned with Michigan educational benchmarks. Wham! Then it hits me. I left Hannah and the family at home this morning (before the majority of them were even up) and off to work I went. Bad Dad. Where are my priorities? What's the important stuff?

As I listen to daily issues of "bathroom time," "laminator protocol," and "school improvement," I find myself thinking of the matter of the moment and in which moment I want to live. You can't just drop out of life and work, but it does make you reevaluate the daily stuff and what it all adds up to. Don't get me wrong. I love being in the classroom and working with kids. They are amazing, caring, young individuals who have their own issues—also known commonly as, "When is snack time?"

Enjoy each moment, hug as much as you can without serving jail time, pray often, change your focus as long as it doesn't endanger your driving skills, and use cool catch phrases whenever possible.

Hannah is beginning to hit her low counts, but unlike the other times, she also has a nasty cough and an arm that requires healing. Yet she still manages to eek out a smile and keeps a positive attitude.

Kazoo Is Not Just for Humming Into

Day 127:
Another day, another hospital room.
We're back.
Seems like we just finished with adjustable beds, food on a tray, cable television that only gets the Dis-

ney Channel, and buzzers that seem to have a mind of their own.

Hannah began with a sniffle that developed into a sniffle, cough, and gradually moved into a sniffle, cough, fever! As her blood counts dropped to a low–low, we were on the go–go. The nearest hospital that can handle the hemoc children of the world is in Kalamazoo, Michigan (famous in a song and known for the land of construction—it's like mini Chicago where construction is concerned).

The doctors are giving us a couple of days of hospital rest, which is ironic since this is the last place you actually rest. The nurses are telling us that we will more than likely be here for the week. What it will come down to is Hannah's counts and how soon they turn around.

As for the nasty fever, it is currently a thing of yesterday. She seems to have broken the downward spiral for now.

Minus the Techno

Day 130:
Take away my technology toys and you're left with me in junior high all over again.

This week was incredibly trying. The DSL is on its way to being installed, but not quite ready. The phone company tried to "hook us up" and ended up "knocking us out" of service. We went for a day and a half with no phone except the outside box. We literally had to go outside to the phone box on the side of the house, open the box, plug in the phone, and then use it. I felt like I should sing the tune from *Green Acres* as I played Oliver on the telephone pole. Then the school switched over its service this week, and we lost all connectivity! And just when you think things can't get worse, my e–mail has been unreachable. Yep, it was truly an *oh, sweet Nelly* moment if ever there was one.

The good stuff of this week was our trip to Kalamazoo. Having Hannah admitted to the hospital was not the same as being at home, but it was reassuring and comforting to know that she was under quality care. Her fever broke, coughing died out, and counts began to rise. As of last night, she's now home and enjoying the stay. She should be well enough to actually be out in public by tomorrow. Who would ever stop to think if his/her child is healthy enough to be out in public?

The other good stuff was that I ate a 1500–calorie slice of cheesecake that was well worth it at the hospital! I chased it with a six hundred–calorie smoothie and am now set for the rest of September when it comes to my caloric intake. Think of all the time I'll save in not having to stop to eat.

Hannah and Kim, along with her mom, Anne, will be heading to Mayo next Wednesday while the boys and I hold down the fort at home. Not quite sure why it's called "the fort" when men are left at home alone. I'd be interested to hear your thoughts on it.

Thanks for your prayers and notes.

More Than a Yard

Day 132:

"Daddy, what are you doing?" were the words I heard after working up a sweat in the backyard.

"I'm trying to build an area of relaxation and gathering," seemed like the reasonable answer at the time.

"But you're destroying our yard! I don't like it at all! " was her disheartened reply as tears welled up in her eyes.

"I'm not destroying our yard. I'm building a place where you and the rest of us can come to sit, talk, hang out, and enjoy."

I got nothing. Just a stare. A disapproving stare.

While I worked on the backyard makeover, Hannah glared at me through the window. I wouldn't classify this as family harmony, but the fact that she can't see the big picture just motivates me to push forward and finish the job. She will like it once it's complete and can see that this is a place made from love, built for relaxation, and time with friends. By the time we're finished, we will have an awesome flowering dogwood beside a spacious deck with a fire pit at one end for nighttime gathering (thanks to Odessa—aka: Randy).

Randy from Rust and Dust created an awesome fire pit that has the words "God Bless You," "Friends, Faith, Family," and "Live, Love, Laugh," which wraps around the rim of the pit so that as the fire glows, the words stand out because they are filled with the light of the embers.

Gather the family, grab the calendar. We're hosting a party—"Chemo Complete '07!"

After this next trip to Mayo, I am hoping Kim will return with the schedule for scans in November so we can plan this shindig! With the help of Grandpa Kelly, Grandpa Zylstra, Van, and Odessa, we hope to knock out this backyard makeover in the next three weeks.

Hannah is doing great! Her health is good, and her attitude even better. She began losing her hair for the second time (although this time is much different from the first). I think it's a sign of character to have to go through losing hair again. She never says much about it though.

I'm anxious to see her straighten her arm all the way. "It really hurts to straighten it," is her answer when I prod her to "let it hang." With her surgery, we not only have to work on finger movement and hand strength but also on having her straighten her arm. I suppose it's just time, similar to chemo, just like radiation, and like surgery—just like everything. I want time to speed up when it comes to results yet slow down when it comes to time spent with Hannah. Why can't I have both?

Peace and prayers.

Second thoughts: I'm amazed at the power of prayer. When someone tells me that they are praying for us and for Hannah, it's as if they've just participated in her battle with cancer. The prayers that have been answered are phenomenal and amazing as we've made this journey. From numbers coming up, to saving her arm, it literally takes my breath away as I look at the people who tell me that they have been praying for Hannah. I'm able to choke out a "thank you" because I'm so overwhelmed knowing prayers are answered according to God's plan. So from our family to your prayers, thank you and praise to our Lord.

Home Alone

Day 136:

It is guy time!

Hannah, Kim, and Grandma are off to Mayo for Hannah's second to last chemo treatment.

I thought it would be easier saying goodbye— *nope, wrong again!* It felt more like letting them down. Despite the fact that I play such a vital role at the hospital when it comes to handing Hannah a glass of water, running to the "parent" refrigerator for a pop for

Kim, or adjusting the volume on the television once Hannah has fallen asleep, being there is just that—I'm there.

Now I'm not there, I'm here. Do I miss the eight–hour trek? After all, there's the wonderful Windy City experience of "honk or lose it," the deer count along the side of the road as you travel through Wisconsin, and the fields of corn as you proceed into Minnesota. Sure, I'll miss it all!

We did our fair share of "I'll miss you" before they left. I just hope the people of Minnesota can carry on without my presence. I ask those in Minnesota to give Hannah hugs and kisses from us back here. We guys will be fine doing guy things—like trying to figure out why there's no food in the fridge and what we can make to eat out of a block of cheese and a quarter bag of Fritos.

DSL Live and in Speed

Day 139:
I had the opportunity to talk with Hannah today at St. Mary's Hospital. "Hello, Daddy!"

I love it when she says that in her young–lady voice. It's that forever reminder that no matter what, I'll always be Daddy, and she'll always be my little girl.

We had a *wonderful chat*—she was a pistol on the phone. With the terrific cell phone reception, I found myself repeating every word four times before she finally got them all. "I'll call you back because I can't hear you very well," she said as I squeaked out a last goodbye before hanging up.

Two minutes...three...five... *Oh, come on,* I thought. *She said she'd call right back!* Not one for waiting by the phone, I dialed again.

"Hello, Daddy!"

"Weren't you calling me *right* back?" I was giving her the benefit of doubt.

"Well, I was going to, but..."

Great! I got the "but." If you get the "but," you might as well concede that you've just reached the bottom of the barrel, the last on the list, the end of the line. Getting the "but" is right up there with arriving at the premier of a long anticipated movie, standing in line for hours, then getting to your seat and finding that the woman in front of you is a throw back to the seventies with a beehive hairdo that would now be classified as a moving tribute to nostalgic heritage. Unfortunately, she has put an end to your viewing pleasure do to its four-foot stature.

After getting over my place in the world of Hannah, I got the run down: things are going good. Oh...that's it. There's no more, I checked. She said, "Things are going good." I had one word for her... *laconic.* Go ahead. Look it up if you must.

I have stories from Kim of room decorating with Daniel, Shanna visiting, and a not–so–pleasant experience as Cara, from the therapy department, took her through a painful therapy session. But from Hannah I get, "Things are good." I was waiting for her to drop the other shoe with an "I'll call you right back."

It was a tough day in the world of *Hannah Montana*. We were hoping to snag some tickets for the concert in December in Grand Rapids, Michigan, but for some strange reason, like "Achy Breaky Heart" catching fire, so has Billy's daughter, and her tickets go within a matter of minutes. Nonetheless, we press on in hopes of becoming groupies and/or stalkers and making it to the concert. Of course, by *we* I'm not referring to the men of the Kelly household. We're more of the distant supporters. The farther we are from the concert and all the preteen and teenage screaming girls, the better.

As Hannah moves into Sunday, she will wrap up the chemo medicine and move into fluids. The best thing that she can do is to stay hydrated. Typically we find ourselves back in the hospital visiting the infusion center on Monday to receive one more big bag of fluids and a dose of Zofran, an anti–nausea medicine. Normally the trip to Michigan would follow, yet this go around, Kim and Hannah have meetings with Dr. Shin, Dr. Bishop, and others to go over the plan from here and to discuss her rehab work for her arm and hand.

Peace and prayers.

Smiles of a Five-Year-Old

Day 140:

I couldn't miss day 140—it's a multiple of seven after all. We all know that seven is the world-renowned lucky number.

I have been pushing forward with the backyard makeover in preparation for the Chemo Complete '07 party. Extra work on the fence makes this one of the most sought after landmarks in the Saint Joseph area, as people slow down enough to shout to me as I work, "What the heck are you doing now?"

I don't think the building of the great pyramids took this much effort. Of course, I was painting today, and if you know me, you know that painting is right up there with creating flower arrangements topping "my things to do" chart. I would rather spend time in line at Disney than painting.

I spoke to the girls earlier today, and Hannah was on a roll (literally) with Shanna and Danielle last night. According to Kim, they went on a teepee rampage in the hospital, spreading sunshine along with toilet paper.

Kim also relayed a very touching moment of a five-year-old-girl with brain tumors. The girls spent some time with her last night, and according to the father, it was the first time in a month that he had seen his daughter smile. *And this is why we are where we are at Mayo.* . Kim said that the dad told her, with tears in his eyes, that she hasn't had a happy moment in a month until now. Being back in Michigan while they are at Mayo doesn't keep me from feeling the same awesomeness that these families felt. It's another example of being touched by such a terrible disease.

I sometimes ask, "Why?", and the five–year–old is the answer I got today.

Kim and I talk about whether we continue our treatments in Minnesota (so far from home) or go to Kalamazoo, which is only an hour away. The bottom line is there are two types of healing: one is physical and the other is a mix of spiritual and emotional. Hannah gets the emotional from those who have been there and the spiritual travels with us (with Pastor Kuddes in the wings). It's something intangible for most. It's wonderful to have people come up to you and say that they are praying for you, but there's something more from someone who has walked the road you travel. That's what we have when we go to Mayo. First comes the drive, then comes the "walk."

So therein lay the question, "Do we travel one more time for chemo or do we stay home?"

As for now, Hannah has some doctor visits early in the week before she gets to head for home. We also hope to solidify our plans for a Chemo Complete '07 party in November. I've done a lot of reading online regarding the cancer journey, and the one crucial element is "the party" once you have completed treatments.

Peace and prayers.

October

Living in Cancer

Day 141:

So I'm standing in the rain at Sam's soccer game. I'm playing the part of coach, although I profess to know very little about soccer. I'm hit, out of the blue, with the thought of my *daughter has cancer*.

I don't have cancer, so I'm not living with it as Hannah is. My experience with cancer is one of caretaker where hers is one of the fighter. It's strange how the feeling washes over you like a tidal wave striking full force on the shoreline. One minute you're coaching a soccer game, the next you're frozen with thoughts of the cancer battle and the wonder of *what's next*.

I can't do anything when it comes to this battle—other than support and pray... and pray some more. Talk about feeling helpless. I'm living *in* cancer.

It surrounds you when you least expect it, and it engulfs you in one gulp just when you think you've reached normal. My normal is no longer. I build a fence and think about cancer. I go grocery shopping and think about cancer. Just when you reach one milestone in the cancer treatments, you have another approaching. It's a pass–fail that you don't want to face, and it's a pass–fail that you can't prepare for mentally or physically. Talk about perspective. I had mine adjusted to living *in* cancer.

Peace and prayers.

Fall Bash

Day 143:

We are heading back to Mayo on the seventeenth of October for Hannah's last treatment. It will be good to finish where we started. Dr. Shin decided that she needs to develop more movement in her arm and hand after seeing her today. According to Kim, he wasn't very happy that her elbow hasn't moved very far when extended. Any movement is good movement, though. They want her back in three weeks to check the progress.

In the meantime, we are in the process of planning the big celebration—Chemo Complete '07!

And We Danced

Day 147:

We had the most wonderful time last night. We went to a wedding where we were able to see half of Kim's side of the family—cousins, aunts, uncles, and those who you think you should know because they look so familiar.

The wedding was very nice and had the most memorable music that I've heard in quite a while—like the theme to *Rocky* as the newly married couple made their way into the reception hall. I thought for a second that having lived the *Rocky* saga this summer on cable that they might have played that for my benefit, but then I realized that there might be more important things at hand besides my need to relive my Mickey experience.

Then came the best moment: as the slow music began I had the chance to walk up to Hannah and ask her to dance with me. Her energy was waning as the night carried on, and I thought she might say no despite my dapper dad appearance, but before I could finish my request for a dance partner, she was on her feet leading me to the floor. As the music played, we adjusted our dance style (because I couldn't hold her correct hand), and we forgot about everyone else around us. It was a moment that has been frozen in my mind. The dance came at just the right time because two songs later Hannah was wiped out and ready to go.

You couldn't take the smile off my face with the kids falling asleep in the back seat as we drove home. I took a glance in Kim's direction as she, too, sat there with a smile paralleling mine. We both knew that it was one of those special moments that you savor.

Six Days

Day 151:
Get more duct tape for car.

That's it in a nutshell. Life should be as simple as my car–repair techniques. When the duct tape begins to fall off, put more on and keep driving. I have a Toyota, so I'm guaranteed five hundred thousand miles, but the body begins to slowly disappear at the ten–year mark (I'm going on year sixteen, so I pretty much have a seat and a steering wheel with a little rust holding the car together around me).

All of that just to say things are going well. Hannah's counts should be moving up by now. She had her last shot this morning and will have her blood drawn tomorrow, and if the counts are good, she can go to school on Friday! Wahoo! I'm off the hook for teaching math to her at home.

Update on the *Hannah Montana* story: tickets were set aside by the manager of the Van Andel Arena for Hannah, a friend, and the two moms. On December sixth it will be Hannah watching Hannah. Excited doesn't even begin to describe the mood for this one.

Backyard makeover 2007 is progressing nicely. *Rust and Dust* is working on the iron gate and fire pit (No, that's not a nickname for Sam and Max. It is an actual designer), while the deck goes vertical this Saturday.

In the meantime, we are off to the land of Vikings next Wednesday.

G and G

Day 155:
Gathering to go.

That seems to be the motto for the week. First we gather, then we go. Planning to be gone a week from the job, school, and home seems to take about a week's worth (maybe more) of planning.

I started throwing things into a bag Saturday. "What are you doing?" Kim asked, as if I were taking my newly cleaned clothes from the wash and hiding them so I wouldn't have to face the piles to be put away.

"Packing. We leave in four days. Why put them into a drawer when I'll be pulling them out again?" I use the same reasoning for not making my side of the bed—the ole *I'll just be getting back in it in less than eighteen hours.*

The same goes for school and schoolwork. As a teacher you have to make plans—a lot of plans—to be gone. It's not like any other job that I know of where you have to have a replacement and leave *specific instructions* for them, as well as anticipate any changes that might occur during the day—like a flood of students who have to go to the bathroom all within a fifteen-minute period of one another.

I've been planning, writing out instructions, and getting work laid out for the past week and a half. Ask any teacher, and they'll more than likely tell you that they would rather come to work feeling lousy than have to write out lesson plans for a substitute.

Hannah left this morning for school with a "Don't forget to find out what work you'll need to do while you're gone" speech from me. Yeah, like a child going through her last round of chemo is really going to be focused on schoolwork, but that was *a parent thing to say*.

That's the hard part of dual worlds. On one side you concern yourself with staying up with the class and the things they are learning; on the other, you just want to get through all the medicine they're pumping into you and wrap up chemo—and maybe have a mini celebration at the hospital while you're at it.

Prayers for Danielle this week as she goes through scans on the seventeenth. Danielle had a tumor

removed from the back of the neck area and finished
with chemo treatments back in April.

Peace and prayers.

The People You Meet

Day 158:
We arrived at the Ronald McDonald House to a mix
of people hanging out in the lobby. Usually the House
has a couple of volunteers to greet and to help you, but
this was more than just a few volunteers.

"What grade are you in?" An elderly man asked.
He approached Hannah as we awaited word on room
availability at the Ronald McDonald House. "Fifth,"
she responded with some hesitation, not really knowing where he was going with this line of questioning.

"Where are you coming from?" the gentleman
asked Hannah with a grin.

"Michigan," Hannah answered. She shot us a
look like she wasn't sure she should be answering his
questions.

"Are you married yet?"

"No." Hannah gave him *the look*.

"Well, that's okay. I heard kids from Michigan
were a little slow." *Bada—bump*.

"Do you know your alphabet?" he said, reaching
into a plastic baggie that held balloons and many other
little trinkets.

"Yeah, I know my alphabet." By this time, a broad smile came across Hannah's face. She had the same kind of look you get right before you get sprayed with water by the magic "sniff my flower" bit.

With his smile growing bigger as well, he pulled out a tiny, three–inch sticker. "Could you read these letters for me?" The sticker had the letters I, Y, Q.

Feeling confident in her academic, three–letter ability, Hannah quickly spouted the letters, "I, Y, Q."

With that, the stage was set. One smooth *thump* of the sticker on Hannah's shirt, the grey–haired, one-liner guy replied with, " Well, I wike que too."

We're in Minnesota, the land of the fifty–two–yard field goal. As we get through the long day of tests and doctor visits, I almost long for the hospital room just to get this last treatment started.

Waiting rooms are okay. After all, I get to people watch. For example, I'm sitting next to a woman, who could easily be my grandmother, only I don't think either of my grandmothers read romance novels. But the important part is that at any moment when I finish writing, I'm going to have a nice conversation with her. I'll find out about her family, why she's here, and learn about her hometown. I'll in turn disclose that I'm an undercover DEA agent looking to bring down the Mayo Cartel. You can't get that kind of interaction in a hospital room. What you do get in the hospital room is crushed ice, a television, and a place to kick your shoes off.

Prayers for a successful chemo round.

Hospital Home

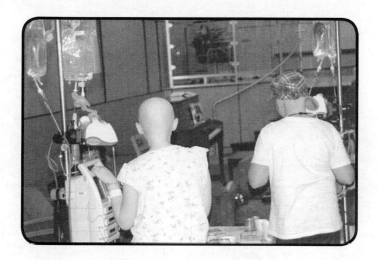

Day 160:

The top ten signs that you know you've spent too much time in the hospital:

10. When you know which rooms on the pediatric floor are the best out of the sixty–seven available.

9. When you know the cleaning lady's routine and get your feet off the floor because the mop is coming.

8. When all conversations begin with talk of medication: "So, what kind of drip do you have going there?"

7. When you can tell the difference between dressing gauzes, and you know which one's the best.

6. When the nurses ask you to give the new parents the tour of the floor.

5. When you go to the pharmacy, and they don't ask for your name anymore.

4. When you not only know the names of all the nurses, but you know their children's names as well.

3. When you find yourself commenting to other kids on the floor: "Say, that's a really nice pole you have."

2. When you begin using the shortcuts between floors that say, "Personnel Only."

1. When you know the Decker family.

When in Mantorville, Buy Candy

Day 162:
Saturday night the chemo countdown was on! You have to pay particular attention to the middle panel of the pump machine as the time ticks. It goes faster than

Dick Clark delivering the New Years Eve rhetoric in Times Square.

We were all thrilled to be on our last drip, but Hannah had one more hookup to go after the chemo bags were packed up and taken away for toxic chemical disposal. Her red blood count wasn't where it should have been, so she was set up for an overnight infusion of blood. As Kim would tell her, "Hope Joe's blood is the good stuff."

All the blood at Saint Mary's Hospital that is used for infusions actually comes directly from the employees. We were told that they feel more confident with the knowledge of their employees' background than with getting blood from a random blood bank. I'm sure we got our blood from a high–ranking Mayo doctor (we have the receipts to prove it was expensive).

Sunday morning, after making the trek to attend church in Waltham, I went to pick up the girls from the hospital, and Hannah was looking *chemo ugly*. Chemo ugly is defined as the last stage on the chemo scale of "how ya feelin'?"

Here, let me break it down for you.

There's chemo fantastic! This is when you're up for visitors; you're able to go on teepee raids; you're able to party Saint Mary's style.

Then there's chemo okay–dokey. This is when you just want to lay around watching television. You're able to have visitors, but they better not stay long. You can play a game as long as it's done at your bedside, and you get to win.

The bottom would be chemo ugly. This is defined simply as "don't talk to me, look at me, or breathe in my presence"; you want nothing to do with anyone. You say, "give me peace; give me quiet. I will puke on you if necessary."

So there we were, right at chemo ugly. We got Hannah back to the RMH, where I proceeded to take a nap (because it was nap time at school—so I'm conditioned for it). By the time I woke up, she had fully recovered and was ready for some chemo complete celebration. Wahoo!

The Hubble House in Mantorville was the first stage of party headquarters for the celebration. With the Decker family on board, we made the drive to the town of Mantorville. However, before we left, Shanna presented Hannah with a very special handcrafted award.

Congrats To Hannah J. Kelly

This award has been presented to a very special girl who has just crossed the finish line in a walk most could never imagine. This girl will forever be an inspiration, and this award is only a small token when compared to the real

gift that our Lord and Savior has given:
a life to live, to enjoy, to cherish
forever, as a gift.

The town of Mantorville had a wonderful treats establishment that would have made the trip worthwhile all by itself, but we had a celebration to start. As always, following chemo, Hannah wanted steak. This was to be Hubble House steak, which anyone from the area would argue would be the only steak to have.

The second stage couldn't have been better selected—the Hucke house (our home away from home and family away from family). We continued the party into the night as the moms took up some fancy Irish dancing, the kids sang their hearts out on karaoke, and the guys settled in for some baseball. Sharing with friends who have been there ahead of us was all we needed at that moment.

All in all, it was a terrific way to celebrate the end of chemo. We look forward to continuing the party in Michigan—and growing hair (just in time for the winter season).

Let's Get Wild

Day 164:
"It's time to get wild on this arm," Dr. Shin said in gusto fashion.

Hannah's eyes couldn't have gotten much larger as Dr. Shin gave her arm and hand the once–over during our visit. Part of her face read *terror*, while the other part smiled at him because you just don't expect your hand surgeon to use those terms. He has such a way with Hannah that, even though he was giving her news with a painful outcome, she had a smile on her face.

Then came Dr. Shives. He walked in and took one look at the stiffness in her elbow and wrist, and came to a similar conclusion. Only instead of "getting wild on that thing," he went with, "we need to start cranking on that." Again Hannah looked with the big eyes at Dr. Shives. I was surprised we didn't need to get an eye doctor in on the action to administer drops to keep her eyes from drying out.

Three words Hannah needs to hear often to get the arm moving, the wrist flexing, and the hand gripping: *push, pull, block.*

She's to work on pushing and pulling both the wrist and elbow, along with bending her fingers (a technique she knows as blocking). The more often she does these three, the better chance we have for future mobility. Doctors want her doing it at least six times a day on her own. However, Hannah has taken this task on like I take on sit–ups—it seems like a good idea.

Peace and prayers.

Hey Now, Hand Lady

Day 171:

That little squirrel in *Over the Hedge* has nothing on fourth graders after a Halloween class party. Having said that, it's good to be back, relaxing and writing. For those who are non–teacher/coaches, it's the end of the quarter (report cards, parent letters, planning, reviewing grades), parent–teacher conferences, basketball tryouts, and practice plans.

Oh yeah, Chemo Complete '07 is closing in fast—and I keep getting confused in the morning between my pants that were pre–chemo days and my pants in post–chemo days (which isn't a great deal of difference if I cared about breathing). Sitting in a hospital room and around various waiting rooms over the course of a summer can take its toll on the waistline.

"Hey, hey, hey, hey, hey!" Hannah's not much for words when it comes to her arm being bent every which way but loose (that's a little something for those Clint fans out there) during physical therapy. It's enough to make you want to wear earplugs, but then there's still the body language and facial expressions that come with it, so earplugs wouldn't help much.

Hannah is on the physical therapy road every day. She's required to work the arm, wrist, and fingers six times a day, but from what we've realized, there's her way of pushing, pulling, and blocking, there's Mom and Dad's way, and then there's the physical therapist's

way. Her arm is starting to show a little bit of movement (which is good), but we have a ways to go before
getting it to zero degrees.

One of her exercises is to take a stack of cups
and work at un–stacking and restacking, in between
stretching up to touch a hand above her head, before
moving on.

We're still working on getting her into a contrap-
tion that will stretch the wrist out and up. The hand
therapists had one ordered, but it didn't seem to do the
job that needs to be done. I'm just glad Dr. Shin isn't
around because I have a feeling he wanted her wrist
stretched already.

Thanks for the prayers. We need mobility soon.

Peace and prayers.

November

Who Needs Hair

Day 173:

Hannah went to school today after getting the all clear on her counts. It was actually picture day for her. Kim said that the photo people stopped by the day before to make sure she was having her photo done today. When I asked Hannah, "Are you going with or without hair?" she proudly responded, "Without, of course."

It's amazing to see how far she has come in six months. The moment she first lost her hair flashed through my mind as she stood before me today, smiling with all that baldness. She was going to have her picture taken naturally. What a difference!

Let the Ball Drop Already

Day 179:

The countdown is on—where's Dick Clark?

I haven't been counting ... *really*. I've been too busy with basketball starting, parent–teacher conferences every night, and planning to be out of class for another four days. There's no time to think about countdowns. That's why I have everyone else doing it for me.

A typical conversation goes something like this:

"Four more days! Are you ready?"

Am I ready? With a look of stunned disbelief on my face, masked quickly with the confidence of Rocky Balboa taking on Clubber Lang, I reply, "Absoluly."

With one day and a wake up (that's a little military jargon for ya—Veteran's Day is coming up), I'm really looking forward to celebrating Chemo Complete '07 with everyone! At the same time, we've been watching our friends via the Internet as they go through their chemotherapy and radiation treatments, keeping them in our prayers. Thousands of children and their families face cancer daily; some are winning the battle and others have already lost. Whether we speak their names or not, we keep them close and celebrate them as well.

Our celebration on Saturday will run right into our departure on Sunday. We head back for Hannah's three-month series of scans and a quick outpatient surgery to remove the port.

Peace and prayers.

Moving Forward

Day 183:

Alive and well.

That simplifies the party–central report.

The party went off without a hitch. Thanks to many special people for stepping up and lending a hand, food, supplies, and organizational skills. We ended up with around 170 at the party to celebrate Chemo Complete '07! Wahoo!

The weather couldn't have been better as we slid the celebration in between a typical November Friday with chilling winds and a wet and gloomy Sunday. Saturday was perfect.

Two days after the celebration: I find myself crammed into the MRI waiting room, lined wall to wall with winter coats and people who are perfecting their winter whooping cough. It's a far cry from the backyard wood–burning, pork–eating, football game–watching, party–going experience just days ago. At various times, I can almost feel the effects of the party, as if I were still there. Perhaps it has something to do with my coat stuffed under my chair, smelling like a nicely stoked fire.

Hannah has tests throughout today with already completing blood draws and the echo cardiogram. The two big ones are her MRI (looking at the forearm) and the CT (checking the lungs). During our meetings with the various doctors, we'll receive the results tomorrow. It's times like these that you take a deep breath and keep your prayer line open.

Prayer for strength to hear the news, prayer for healing and health.

Thanks again for the wonderful opportunity to share this journey.

Peace and prayers.

Flu–Shot Tuesday

Day 184:

"Mom, my stomach feels sick," Hannah said, as we sat in the waiting room this morning waiting for our name to be called.

Today was "result day." After a day of scans and tests yesterday, it all comes down to the first words spoken by the doctor this morning. Would it be, "There are spots on the scans that give us cause to believe ... " or "scans are clear"?

"I'm so nervous," Hannah mutters again. "I don't want to get a flu shot."

Flu shot? That's what has got her worked up? Here we are, on the verge of our first scan results after treatments, and she's concerned about another shot.

"Is the needle long? Will it hurt? I heard it hurts," she said.

Hannah Kelly. Finally, the name is spoken, and we're out of the waiting area and into the room—for more waiting. But, it's progress nonetheless.

Dr. Laack was to be our first doctor visit. It couldn't have been a more appropriate placement in the line up because Dr. Laack was the one who always had a way of telling us the positives during a time when they were hard to come by.

A soft knock at the door (a courtesy before anyone enters the room). Dr. Laack walked into the room with a big smile, handing out hugs all around before we settled back into our seats to hear the news. "Scans look good," she said with a big broad smile. Kim shot from the bench seat for one more *extra* hug from Dr. Laack. You could feel the air as we all took one large exhale. Clear scans—thank God!

After a brief visit with Dr. Laack (and finding out that she was relevantly named Nadia—meaning *hope*), Donna (oncology PA) came into the room to give us the oncology review of the results.

It took Hannah a matter of minutes before she went right back to focusing on the flu shot. I suppose it just goes to show you that no matter what life-threatening challenges you face, flu shots still hold the top rank of things to be concerned about.

Donna went into quick action and set up the shot right then and there. "No time like now!" Donna announced. She knew Hannah wouldn't relax and celebrate the good news until this flu shot was nothing but a memory and a small bump on her leg. The whole thing lasted a mere couple of seconds, with a brief "ouch!" from Hannah.

Tomorrow we have port removal, followed by hand therapy, and Dr. Shin's/Dr. Shives' tag team as they give us a little look into the "what now" portion in dealing with Hannah's disability. It'll be another full day, but with the weight of the scan results off of our shoulders, it will be a piece of cake. Oh yeah, and the fact that the flu shot is now a memory for 365 more days, it's all wonderful.

Peace and prayers.

See You In

Day 186:
Five words are all it took to make a grin reach from ear to ear: *"See you in three months."*

We are free and clear for the next three months. That gives us time to grow hair, unbend an arm, build strength, enjoy the holidays, settle into school, and dream of purchasing a new car for the next ten years or more of travel to Mayo.

Dr. Shives and Dr. Shin were both pleased with the progress that Hannah had made with her movement. Yet, it was what Dr. Laack told us that reverberates in our thoughts: "Don't let the scar tissue get ahead of you." Hannah needs to continually work her arm and massage her scars for the next year (as the scar tissue continues to try and take hold).

The plan: Over the next few years, Hannah will need scans every three months to check her lungs and arm. The chance of recurrence to her arm is lower than it metastasizing to the lungs. Dr. Laack told us that if it's going to recur in the arm, it typically shows itself within the first two years. However, there's always a chance.

Prayers for a little boy named Silas. He has been fighting an aggressive neuroblastoma since January 2007. He recently was released from Mayo, and while at home, went to the doctor with his dad, Randy, for a small cough. While having a chest X–ray done to look for pneumonia, they found spots on his lungs. He and his parents are back at Mayo again and the neuroblastoma has resurfaced. We know the power of prayer firsthand, and this family needs all the power we can give them.

Peace and prayers.

December and Beyond

Scan Forward

I know it is supposed to be a comfort when the doctor tells you, "We'll see you in three months for check ups," but it's not really.

"I feel sick to my stomach," Kim informs me as we head back to Minnesota for our second after–treatment scans. The nine–hour drive gives you a great deal of time to sit and think.

Trying to rationalize Kim's fears, I offered, "I think it has a lot to do with the fact that we are no longer shooting her up with drugs or radiation to combat any possible microscopic cancer cells, and we're left to deal with the 'we hope we got it all' aspect." There I went again, trying to break things down logically, when all she needed to hear was that I was nervous as well.

I could tell by the look on her face that I missed the target once again. The look she gave me said, "Just drive and say comforting things every now and then." Kim closed her eyes to pass the time and miles. The kids were in the back of the van enjoying a movie on the portable DVD player.

Scans are a double–edged sword. On one hand you look forward to getting the body scanned and checked out to hear those reassuring words of, "We have clear scans." Those are the words of celebration, the words of another three months of life, the words that make you want to go eat some wings!

Yet, there remains too often those feelings of recurrence and the possibility that this battle may not be over just yet. *What if the scans come back with cancer? Have we done everything right to this point?* As a family dealing with cancer, you often see others who have come back to fight a second time.

I'm reminded of meeting a fellow father at the Ronald McDonald House.

"This is our second time fighting this," said the farmer from North Dakota, as we stood in the kitchen of the House. "He had experienced headaches when he was eight. Turned out to be brain tumors. We took care of it then and thought it was over. Now he's eighteen, and we're back again. It wasn't more than two weeks ago, when he had two jobs and was completing high school."

It's stories like these that add to your anxiety. You've already been down the rocky road of cancer treatments. Why is there a need to relive it? "Trust in the Lord with all your heart and lean not on your own understanding" (Proverbs 3:5, NIV). It's that simple, but does this help? Heck no, it doesn't! We're human after all. We worry when we know worrying doesn't help. We raise anxiety to the maximum when we know we have no control. We admit we hold no power greater than that of God, but it doesn't stop us from mentally diving into the pool of doubt. *Snap out of it!*

Thanks for reading.

Peace and prayers.

Get Your Cookies!

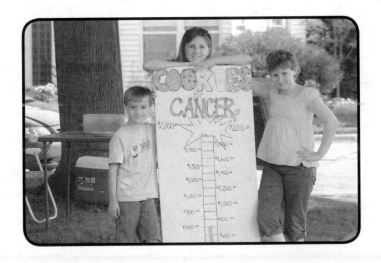

It's amazing what a lemonade/cookie stand can raise in a three-hour period. "Hannah, how did you do?" I asked. I was curious what the effect of a cookie stand had when placed directly across the street from the little league hot dog stand.

Let me back up for a moment.

Location, location, location. Our home is directly across from three youth baseball fields. In the months of May and June these are packed with loving, screaming, cheering grandparents/parents and siblings.

Hannah and her friend, Emily, decided to set up a lemonade/cookie stand yesterday . As they prepared to go head–to–head with the hot dog stand that the league runs, my mind envisioned the commissioner of the league making his way to my front door to discuss the situation.

I opened up the conversation. "Hannah, I don't think this is such a good idea." She and Emily laid out the treats on the table, which had now turned my front lawn into a storefront of goodies.

"Dad, we did it last year!" She firmly reminded me of last year's success with the lemonade stand in May—prior to our leaving for Mayo.

"Yes, but you were selling lemonade during practice times when the concession stand was closed. They're open now, and I don't think they will like the fact that you're taking their customers away."

"Well, they don't sell lemonade or cookies, so it doesn't matter," she retorted with the confidence of a DECCA member. It's all about the market!

I still wasn't feeling really comfortable as I worked in the backyard, listening to the girls in the front give their sales cry—"Cookies…lemonade!"—to each passing pedestrian.

After about an hour, I checked the progress, and I must say, it wasn't just the average lemonade/cookie stand. The girls had decided to raise money for kids with cancer and animals at the Humane Society. They had taken news clippings that had Hannah's story and photos and placed them on the table to share with those who stopped. Along with separate buckets for a collection point, the girls had labels designated for Cancer Kids and Humane Society.

Later that night, Kim and I had one of those talks, the kind where you're really tired and don't feel much like talking, but when a good thing happens, you just have to stay up and talk it through.

"What do you think about this cookie idea?" I asked, already knowing the answer. If we agreed to continue and support Hannah with this quest, it would mean that Kim would be spending a great deal of her time assisting in the production. Not to be biased or anything, but she does make the best cookies around.

"I think it's a fantastic idea," was her reply.

Oh, sweet Nelly. Cookies could be the beginning to OSN (Oncology Societal Network). Sell a cookie, share a story, and by the way, would you care for a lemonade to wash it down with?

The next morning I asked, "Hannah, how did you do?" and waited to hear the results.

"Twenty seven dollars and two cents," was her matter–of–fact reply.

We're off and running. Hannah and friends have made it a mission to raise money for children who are having treatments for cancer. (The money for the Humane Society would have to be placed on hold for now.)

Chew On This

We were already running short on cookies!

I dialed Kim's phone and impatiently waited for her to answer. Finally she picked up.

"Where are you?'

"I'm at the store. Hey, I have nine missed calls. Was that you?" Kim's response seemed a little less frantic than what I had hoped for.

"Yes! That would have been me trying to reach you." We were in the beginning of the Cookies for Cancer Kids and already running short on product. Kim had planned on baking a few more batches, but the fact that we had not checked the egg supply left our ingredients a bit lacking. Chef Ramsey would not have been happy.

Yesterday, Hannah had a great day as the community rolled up to the front of our house for cookies, lemonade, and a chance to speak with Hannah, thanks to an article in the local paper, MailMax. I, of course, was banned from the cookie area for no particular reason other than, "Dad, here come some people. You need to go now." Hannah put it to me in a matter-of-fact manner. I can only assume that she felt that if I were there, they would want to talk to me instead of her handling things herself. Fair enough. I became the runner man (run for this, run for that).

When the whole family got rolling, we made quite the team. Even Sam and Dustin (my nephew) decided to jump into the cookie-making experience. We will add the disclaimer, though, that we did not sell any of their creations. Yet, surprisingly enough, the lumped together cookie of mush was very tasty.

Hannah, along with the assistance of Max and Lilly (my niece), doubled their June sales in one day. Hannah already has plans to purchase books, games, and crafts for the children.

Someone did ask for her hours. Good question! It's been during baseball games up to this point, but they wrap-up with the league this week, so we'll have to put some thought to this question and get back to everyone. We've talked about it, and she would like to continue.

What Are You Waiting For? Pop a Top!

It's difficult to sit back and not do something, particularly when doing something benefits those who come after you in the cancer walk. With our experience at the Ronald McDonald House, we have a deeper appreciation for what is done to support families who need to worry about nothing else but their child. Hannah has decided to add collecting pop–tops for the Ronald McDonald House to her cookie stand.

We set out to create a DVD that she could share with local schools, but what we eventually found out is that they already have a pop–top collection in place. Does everyone have one of these in their community? If not, they should because it is such an easy way to help support others.

We still made the DVD (partly because it was just fun to make), which she played for those stopping to buy a cookie and drink lemonade. The collection process was still on track though. "We can still collect at the stand and at my school," Hannah commented.

If you have a pop can and nowhere to put that top you just popped off out of boredom, – rinse it, store it, and give Hannah a call—she's ready to collect a couple million!

Peace and prayers.

Becoming United

The United Way has asked Hannah to be one of their speakers this year. Through the Berrien County Cancer Service (which receives support and funding from the United Way), Hannah was able to receive blood draws through her port rather than her arm (which just resulted in a lot of crying and several attempts to find a vein). Our nurse, Connie, would come right to the house to draw blood from the port, which in turn gave us the count information we needed. Before we were told about Connie, we had to travel to Kalamazoo because no one in this area had the training to access a child's port. I know. Strange, huh? But that's what we were told.

"Aren't you coming with me?" Hannah asked. She was about to give her first United Way speech as she walked toward the UPS drivers standing in the middle of the warehouse floor.

The drivers had been trickling in for the past thirty minutes as we stood by with our United Way representative, Retta. All dressed in their customary brown, they strolled through the door to take their place among the other drivers at the end of the open bay.

"Okay, we're ready to get started. I'll gather the drivers for stretching first." Brooke, the foreman, told us as he motioned us to follow him. Who knew that the drivers warmed up before they hit the streets? I would have been even more impressed had they performed a little two–mile run. "Let's go. Everyone circle around for stretching!"

Following the stretching and a brief announcement, Retta stepped forward with Hannah (in the middle of the sea of brown) and gave her talk on how the United Way assists in our area. Then she introduced Hannah.

Hannah doesn't have a projective voice just yet, which caused the brown circle to close in tighter around her as they tried to hear her over the noises associated with a package delivery warehouse. I saw the same scene in the *Lion King* with the hyenas—only the drivers were way nicer, and rather than pounce, they gave Hannah applause when she finished.

"Well, what did you think?" I asked. I was anxious to hear how she felt about the experience.

"They made me nervous when they all moved in! But, it was fun." She had that smile on her face that clearly said, "Yes, I did it!"

One down, more to go. "Are you busy tomorrow?" Retta asked. She had another company in mind for Hannah to talk to.

Never Alone

Childhood cancer, along with all other cancers, is something that no family should have to go through alone. Thanks for the tremendous support, prayers, and uplifting way others have reached out to our family.

There are a number of organizations out there that make it their business to support families going through childhood cancer. Be sure to contact your social worker at your hospital or clinic and ask for help. You won't know what to ask for, and that's okay. They know what you need.

A year out of treatments, and we are still finding groups like Brighter Tomorrows to be a source of strength, hope, and information for our family.

Thanks for reading.

Peace and prayers and the end to cancer as we know it.

> We also rejoice in our sufferings, because we know that suffering produces perseverance; perseverance, character, and character, hope. And hope does not disappoint us, because God has poured out His love into our hearts by the Holy Spirit, whom He has given us.
>
> Romans 5:3–6 (NIV)

listen|imagine|view|experience

AUDIO BOOK DOWNLOAD INCLUDED WITH THIS BOOK!

In your hands you hold a complete digital entertainment package. Besides purchasing the paper version of this book, this book includes a free download of the audio version of this book. Simply use the code listed below when visiting our website. Once downloaded to your computer, you can listen to the book through your computer's speakers, burn it to an audio CD or save the file to your portable music device (such as Apple's popular iPod) and listen on the go!

How to get your free audio book digital download:

1. Visit www.tatepublishing.com and click on the e|LIVE logo on the home page.
2. Enter the following coupon code:
   fbd8-e1a8-5d5c-205b-9631-b1c5-115a-e136
3. Download the audio book from your e|LIVE digital locker and begin enjoying your new digital entertainment package today!